Pigmentation Disorders - Etiology and Recent Advances in Treatments

Edited by Shahin Aghaei

Published in London, United Kingdom

Pigmentation Disorders - Etiology and Recent Advances in Treatments
http://dx.doi.org/10.5772/intechopen.100979
Edited by Shahin Aghaei

Contributors
Nayra Merino, Maria Eugenia Gaviño, Marta García-Bustinduy, Mónica Fumero, Donnell J. Creel, Ivan Arni C. Preclaro, Emine Müge Acar, Anita Damodaran, Nirmala Nair, Fatimata Ly, Behrooz Kasraee, Shahin Aghaei, Ali Moradi, Ana Paula da Silva Urzedo, Marisa Gonzaga Da Cunha

First published in London, United Kingdom, 2023 by IntechOpen
IntechOpen is the global imprint of INTECHOPEN LIMITED, registered in England and Wales, registration number: 11086078, 5 Princes Gate Court, London, SW7 2QJ, United Kingdom

British Library Cataloguing-in-Publication Data
A catalogue record for this book is available from the British Library

Additional hard and PDF copies can be obtained from orders@intechopen.com

Pigmentation Disorders - Etiology and Recent Advances in Treatments
Edited by Shahin Aghaei
p. cm.
Print ISBN 978-1-80356-899-7
Online ISBN 978-1-80356-900-0
eBook (PDF) ISBN 978-1-80356-901-7

Meet the editor

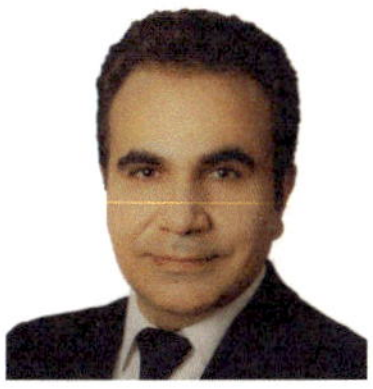

Shahin Aghaei, MD, graduated from Shiraz University of Medical Sciences, Shiraz, Iran, in 2004. He was awarded a dermatopathology fellowship at Charles University in Prague, Czech Republic, in 2008 by the International Society of Dermatology, followed by a dermatological surgery fellowship at the Medical University of Graz, Austria, in 2010. He is currently an associate professor of dermatology and dermatologic surgery at the School of Medicine, Iran University of Medical Sciences, Tehran, Iran. He is editor-in-chief of the *Journal of Surgical Dermatology* in Singapore. He is a member of the American Academy of Dermatology (AAD), European Academy of Dermatology and Venereology (EADV), American Society for Laser Medicine and Surgery (ASLMS), International Society of Dermatology (ISD), International Hyperhidrosis Society, and Iranian Society of Dermatology.

Contents

Preface

Pigmentation disorders affecting the patient's skin color are relatively common diseases in skin clinics. The skin gets its color from a pigment called melanin, which is produced by special cells in the skin called melanocytes. When melanocytes are damaged or unhealthy, melanin production is disrupted. Generally, pigmentation disorders can be divided into two groups: hyperpigmented and hypopigmented. In hyperpigmented conditions, there is an increase in melanin production. Melasma, age spots, and post-inflammatory hyperpigmentation are common examples of these disorders. Hyperpigmented conditions can be caused by skin damage, burns, exposure to sunlight, pregnancy, hormone therapy, and other skin diseases such as acne.

When the body cannot produce enough melanin, the skin loses its color partially or completely. Hypopigmentation conditions can be caused by genetic factors, immunological changes, trauma, and inflammation, as well as blisters, burns, dermatitis, and fungal infections. One such disorder, vitiligo, causes white, non-scaly patches on the skin, especially on the skin of elbows, knees and periorificial areas such as around the eyes and mouth.

This book contains nine chapters in five sections which discuss the latest findings and treatments of the most common skin pigment diseases. Section 1, "Hyperpigmentation Disorders", opens with a chapter on melasma, a common hyperpigmentation disorder that is classified based on brown pigmentation in sun-exposed areas such as the face. Extensive courses of treatment, which are often quite problematic, are required for stable maintenance care As it involves exposed areas of the face, melasma can have a severe impact on a patient's quality of life and causes emotional, psychological, and social stress. Melasma is usually more common in women with higher phototypes (III–V). It can be triggered by pregnancy, contraceptives, thyroid disease, hormone therapy and exposure to sunlight. Chapter 2 explores the pathogenic mechanism of melasma and reviews treatments.

The two chapters in Section 2, "Hypopigmentation Disorders", examine the pathogenesis, clinical features, treatment, and psychological impact of vitiligo, a condition that affects 0.5–2% of the population worldwide. Selective loss of melanocytes is a characteristic feature of vitiligo. Among the many theories proposed for melanocyte loss, the convergence theory, which suggests that a combination of biochemical, environmental, and immunological factors play a role in the pathophysiology of vitiligo, is currently the most widely accepted theory. Treatment options, depending on the subtype, extent, distribution and activity of the disease, include local and systemic immunosuppressants, phototherapy, and surgery. Psychological conditions associated with vitiligo include stigma, adjustment disorders, sleep disturbance, relationship problems including sexual dysfunction, and avoidant or restrictive behavior. Depression, anxiety and alexithymia have also been reported. Female gender, visible or genital lesions, age less than 30 years, and more involvement of the body surface are risk factors for developing mental illnesses. Psychological tests (HADS, TAS-20, DLQI, or BDI-II) can be useful to evaluate these patients and decide on a better treatment approach.

Section 3, "Medications and Pigmentation Disorders", opens with an overview of the most significant skin pigmentation molecules used in hyperpigmentation treatments. The most effective depigmenting agents, such as hydroquinone and the Kligman formula, are associated with long-term side effects, but safer depigmenting agents, such as kojic acid, arbutin, and niacinamide, may be less effective. Tranexamic acid and cysteamine are two new and interesting molecules that seem to fulfill most of the required properties of an acceptable skin-whitening agent. Drug-induced pigmentation occurs in 20% of skin pigment disorders. Its occurrence has been reported in certain drugs, including alkylating/cytotoxic agents, analgesics, antiarrhythmics, anticoagulants, antiepileptics, antimalarials, antimicrobials, antiretrovirals, metals, prostaglandin analogs, and psychotropic agents. The proposed mechanisms include (1) melanin accumulation, (2) drug accumulation, (3) new pigment production, and (4) iron deposition. Although drug association is difficult to confirm, history, with an emphasis on medications currently being used, and clinical examination, may guide clinicians to an accurate diagnosis. Treatment options include drug discontinuation, adequate sun protection, and non-ablative pigment lasers. The final chapter in this section reviews prominent hyperpigmentation manifestations such as post-inflammatory hyperpigmentation (e.g., acne-related), solar lentigo, melasma, and periorbital hyperpigmentation, together with recent advances in aesthetic interventions.

Section 4 is titled "Pigmentation Disorders in Skin of Color". Pigment disorders are more frequently seen in patients with darker phototypes (Fitzpatrick IV to VI). Inflammatory dermatoses such as acne are often associated with hyperpigmentation after inflammation, but psoriasis and lichen planus are associated with dyschromia. Some skin diseases such as mycosis fungoides have unusual manifestations in the form of hypopigmented plaques. All of these dyschromias have a significant impact on quality of life and are responsible for practices such as voluntary cosmetic depigmentation with products such as steroids, hydroquinone, mercury salts, and various depigmentation products. This procedure is the source of pigment disorders such as exogenous ochronosis, lichenoid and lupoid dermatoses, and hyperpigmentation around the eyes. For this reason, treatment management is difficult, so early diagnosis of the disease and appropriate treatment are recommended.

Section 5, "The Role of Melanin in Internal Organs", discusses the role of melanin pigment in the retina and inner ear. Melanin pigment is normally present in the outermost layer of the retina, in the inner ear adjacent to capillaries in stria vascularis near hair cells, and in vestibular organs. Significant reduction in melanin pigment in mammals is associated with embryonic miswiring and disruption of visual and auditory function. The consequences for the visual system include abnormal development of the retina and misrouting of optic pathways into the brain impairing visual acuity, eye movement and stereovision. Lack of melanin pigment in the inner ear is associated with greater susceptibility to noise damage and poorer localization of sound in space.

I would like to thank the editorial team at IntechOpen for their kind help and support with the publication of this book.

Shahin Aghaei, MD
Department of Dermatology and Dermatological Surgery,
School of Medicine,
Iran University of Medical Sciences,
Tehran, Iran

Section 1

Hyperpigmentation Disorders

Chapter 1

Introductory Chapter: Quality of Life in the Patients with Melasma

Shahin Aghaei and Ali Moradi

1. Introduction

When we were thinking about the title for the introductory chapter, naturally, the most common pigmentation diseases were the priority [1]. In other chapters of the book, vitiligo was discussed from both psychological and clinical aspects. On the other hand, the clinical course of melasma and post-inflammatory hyperpigmentation was present in other chapters, but there was no room for a psychological discussion of melasma patients and its effects on the patient's quality of life.

Melasma is a characteristic pattern of marginated facial hyperpigmentation, occurring primarily on the face. The cause of melasma is not completely known, but pregnancy, estrogen therapy, exposure to sunlight and ultraviolet light, and positive family history in Caucasian patients are well known [2]. Melasma is more common in women and non-Caucasian people, although it has been seen in men of all races [2, 3].

Melasma can have significant emotional and psychological impacts on patients. The 10-item the *Melasma Quality of Life (MELASQOL)* scale was devised from the comprehensive Health-Related Quality of Life (HRQoL) assessment set [4, 5]. HRQoL is a scale used to define the social, physical, and psychological well-being of an individual and to evaluate the distress of disease on daily living [6, 7].

In this chapter, we will concisely review the clinical aspects, treatments, and the impact of melasma on the quality of life (QoL) of the patients.

2. Clinical manifestations

Melasma is an acquired hyperpigmentation ailment in which some light to dark brown and irregular macules and patches are distributed on the sunlight-exposed body areas. Lesions are usually on the skin of the forehead, temples, upper lip, and cheeks [8].

It is often disseminated in one of four clinical patterns, that is, centrofacial, malar, mandibular, and extrafacial; the last pattern is variable but is predominantly located on the upper extremities, often on sun-exposed sites. It is known that the centrofacial pattern is the most common type. Melasma is sometimes classified as epidermal, dermal, or mixed types based on the level of melanin deposition in the epidermis and/or the dermis [2, 9].

The disorder is common in women, especially during reproductive ages, although it is possible in the teenage years, in older women who take special medicines, and sometimes in men [10]. Although the main cause of melasma is still unknown, it seems to be the result of genetic and environmental factors that play a role in causing it [4].

Among the many factors that are associated with melasma, contact with sunlight is the most related [8]. Among other factors, pregnancy, some hormones, birth control pills, some endocrine disorders, especially thyroid gland disorders, family history, using some cosmetic products, anti-epileptics, and phototoxic drugs are seen [11, 12].

Wood's lamp is a simple diagnostic device that can be used to see the depth of skin pigmentation. When exposed to UV light in a dark environment, the pigmented skin is clearly visible, and the dark border becomes fluorescent [13]. Moreover, with Wood's lamp, superficial or epidermal melasma is usually seen more clearly under light, whereas deep or dermal melasma shows no particular changes [14].

When examined with a dermoscope, in superficial or epidermal melasma, a network of brown reticulated islands with dark and small seeds can be seen scattered [14]. Reflectance confocal microscopy can be used in cellular evaluation in patients with melasma. Sometimes a skin biopsy is used to confirm the diagnosis of melasma and of course often to rule out other differential diagnoses.

3. Treatments

The most common therapeutic agents used are those that inhibit the production of melanin by decreasing melanogenesis and melanocyte proliferation. Using 2–5% hydroquinone cream at night for 2 to 4 months has a significant improvement in melasma. Kojic acid, azelaic acid, and tranexamic acid can be mentioned as topical treatments. In the treatment of melasma, before using chemical peeling or laser therapy, it is better to use only topical treatments first [15]. Kligman's formula, which is a mixture of hydroquinone, tretinoin, and dexamethasone in a cream base, is currently the best treatment for melasma and leads to recovery in 60–80% of patients, which is why it is called the gold standard treatment [9, 16, 17]. The use of hats and broad-spectrum sunblock creams is very important for the success of melasma treatment and the prevention of the recurrence of the disease.

Oral tranexamic acid has become popular because of its low price and availability. A meta-analysis study of randomized controlled trials shows that this drug has significant efficacy and safety [18]. But before prescribing it, the physician should consult with the patient about the dosage and its side effects. It should be noted that topical use of tranexamic acid has no significant effect.

The use of chemical peels and lasers should be approached with caution, as they may exacerbate or cause a relapse of melasma [9]. These interventions should be undertaken by an expert with an understanding of skin color. A series of 3–6 sessions of chemical peels with active ingredients, such as alpha hydroxy acids (AHA), for example, 6–12% glycolic acid cream or lotion, and beta hydroxy acids (BHA), for example, salicylic acid, has also been shown to be useful in the treatment of melasma as they can remove surface skin and decrease the physiological activity of tyrosinase [19].

Intense pulsed light (IPL) devices have a range of different wavelengths that are used to treat superficial and deep melasma [20]. This treatment is better used together at the same time with topical medications. IPL treatment only gives a moderate improvement if it is not combined with topical treatments, and the recurrence rate will also be moderate. Q-switched lasers, ablation lasers, and picosecond lasers can also be used to treat melasma but may cause deeper hyperpigmentation after treatment [9, 20].

In general, laser therapy, compared to topical treatments, has a higher probability of recurrence and disease resistance to treatment [9]. Some treatments may be associated with post-inflammatory hyperpigmentation or hypopigmentation, which should be considered before treatment. Cosmetic camouflage creams can be an important auxiliary treatment for these complications in patients [17].

Finally, it is important to mention that the treatment of melasma should often be done with a multifaceted approach, and its goal is to reduce pigment production and achieve balance in the patient's skin [16]. Because of the high chance of recurrence, maintenance treatments are often required, along with protection from strong sunlight with broad-spectrum sunscreens.

4. Quality of life

Despite the existence of various drugs and methods in the treatment of melasma, there is little information about their effect on the daily lives of patients. Health-related quality of life (HRQoL) is a measure to describe a person's physical, social, and mental health and assess the disease burden in daily life [6, 7]. When a patient has extensive melasma on the face, a person's overall emotional health can be significantly affected, also leading to reduced social functioning, efficiency at work or school, and decreased self-confidence [6, 7, 21].

As melasma has a much impact on the psychological aspects of a patient's life than on the physical, a new instrument was needed to more accurately determine the HRQoL in these patients [4].

Some studies have shown that the three life domains most affected by melasma are social life, recreation and leisure, and emotional well-being. The sensitivity to change of the MELASQOL was examined in 72.8% of the patients with melasma. These patients were reassessed 6–8 months following topical treatment and demonstrated highly significant improvement in the MELASQOL total score. The largest effect size was obtained in the social life domain. These results indicate that MELASQOL is able to capture changes in patients' improvement that are not reflected in clinical rating scales of melasma severity. In addition, the present studies provide evidence for the excellent responsiveness of MELASQOL to treatment-induced changes [4, 5].

As mentioned before, melasma occurs in exposed areas of the body, especially in the face, and clearly affects the appearance of sufferers, so the patient is affected by the mental aspects and social illness, and almost always it affects the generality of the patients and has an effect on the quality of life of the sufferers that results in the influence of a person's self-concept and the patient's self-confidence [22]. Melasma is also due to people's complaints about their appearance and beauty, which causes many problems. It creates an obvious psychological problem in patients [12, 23].

Measuring the quality of life in skin diseases is very important because these diseases are not mostly life-threatening [12], but through different ways, such as causing symptoms (itching and pain), mental pressure (deficiency of self-confidence and nervousness), influence on social relations and family, and treatment problems (financial burden and waste of time), they can affect the patient's life [24, 25].

Melasma is no exception to this rule; the results of the studies carried out indicate that melasma is very destructive to the quality of life of the sufferers and has the most negative effect in the areas of social life, entertainment, and mental health of patients' lives [23, 26].

5. Conclusions

Melasma has a significant negative impact on the patient's quality of life. Thus, evaluating the quality of life of patients with melasma during treatment should not be ignored. Additionally, utilization of the DLQI and especially the MELASQoL scale should be considered in the care plan.

Competing interest

None declared.

Author details

Shahin Aghaei[1*] and Ali Moradi[2]

1 Department of Dermatology, School of Medicine, Iran University of Medical Sciences, Tehran, Iran

2 School of Medicine, Semmelweis University, Budapest, Hungary

*Address all correspondence to: shahinaghaei@yahoo.com

References

[1] Dlova NC, Akintilo LO, Taylor SC. Prevalence of pigmentary disorders: A cross-sectional study in public hospitals in Durban, South Africa. International Journal of Women's Dermatology. 2019;**5**:345-348

[2] Sanchez NP, Pathak MA, Sato S. Melasma: A clinical, light microscopic, ultrastructural, and immunofluorescence study. Journal of the American Academy of Dermatology. 1981;**4**:698-710

[3] McDonald CJ. Dermatological problems in black skin. Program Dermatology. 1973;**4**:10-20

[4] Balkrishnan R, McMichael AJ, Camacho FT, Saltzberg F, Housman TS, Grummer S, et al. Development and validation of a health-related quality of life instrument for women with melasma. The British Journal of Dermatology. 2003;**149**(3):572-577

[5] Aghaei S, Moradi A, Mazharinia N, Abbasfard Z. The melasma quality of life scale (MELASQOL) in Iranian patients: A reliability and validity study. Journal of the European Academy of Dermatology and Venereology. 2005;**19**(suppl.2):39

[6] Anderson RT, Rajagopalan R. Development and validation of a quality of life instrument for cutaneous diseases. Journal of the American Academy of Dermatology. 1997;**37**:41-50

[7] Finlay AY. Quality of life measurement in dermatology: A practical guide. The British Journal of Dermatology. 1997;**136**:305-314

[8] Victor FC, Gelber J, Rao B. Melasma: A review. Journal of Cutaneous Medicine and Surgery. 2004;**8**:97-102

[9] Oakley A, Doolan BJ, Gupta M. Melasma. Hamilton, NZ: DermNet NZ, 2020; 2020. Available from: dermnetnz.org/topics/melasma. [Accessed: November 20, 2022]

[10] Jadotte YT, Schwartz RA. Melasma: Insights and perspectives. Acta Dermatovenerologica Croatica. 2010;**18**:124-129

[11] Damoa AS, Lambert WC, Schwartz RA. Melasma: Insight into a distressing dyschromia. Anais Brasileiros de Dermatologia. 2014;**89**(5):771-782

[12] Cestari TF, Hexsel D, Viegas ML, et al. Validation of a melasma quality of life questionnaire for Brazilian Portuguese language: The MelasQol-BP study and improvement of Qol of melasma patients after triple combination therapy. The British Journal of Dermatology. 2007;**156**(suppl. 1):13-20

[13] Ponka D, Baddar F. Wood lamp examination. Canadian Family Physician. 2012;**58**(9):976

[14] Sonthalia S, Jha AK, Langar S. Dermoscopy of melasma. Indian Dermatology Online Journal. 2017;**8**(6):525-526. DOI: 10.4103/idoj.IDOJ_6_17

[15] Grimes PE, Ijaz S, Nashawati R, Kwak D. New oral and topical approaches for the treatment of melasma. International Journal Women's Dermatology. 2018;**5**(1):30-36. DOI: 10.1016/j.ijwd.2018.09.004

[16] Sarma N, Chakraborty S, Poojary SA, et al. Evidence-based review, grade of recommendation, and suggested treatment recommendations for melasma. Indian Dermatology Online

Journal. 2017;**8**(6):406-442. DOI: 10.4103/idoj.IDOJ_187_17

[17] Rodrigues M, Pandya AG. Melasma: Clinical diagnosis and management options. The Australasian Journal of Dermatology. 2015;**56**(3):151-163. DOI: 10.1111/ajd.12290

[18] Feng X, Su H, Xie J. Efficacy and safety of tranexamic acid in the treatment of adult melasma: An updated meta-analysis of randomized controlled trials. Journal of Clinical Pharmacy and Therapeutics. 2021;**46**(5):1263-1273. DOI: 10.1111/jcpt.13430

[19] Sharad J. Glycolic acid peel therapy—A current review. Clinical, Cosmetic and Investigational Dermatology. 2013;**6**:281-288. DOI: 10.2147/CCID.S34029

[20] Trivedi MK, Yang FC, Cho BK. A review of laser and light therapy in melasma. International Journal of Women's Dermatology. 2017;**3**(1):11-20. DOI: 10.1016/j.ijwd.2017.01.004

[21] Aghaei S, Sodaifi M, Jafari P, Mazharinia N, Finlay AY. DLQI scores in vitiligo reliability and validity of the Persian version. BMC Dermatology. 2004;**4**:8

[22] Balkrishnan R, McMichael AJ, Hu JY, et al. Correlates of health-related quality of life in women with severe facial blemishes. International Journal of Dermatology. 2006;**45**:111-115

[23] Dominguez AR, Balkrishnan R, Ellzey AR, Pandya AG. Melasma in Latina patients: Cross cultural adaptation and validation of a quality-of-life questionnaire in Spanish language. Journal of the American Academy of Dermatology. 2006;**55**:59-66

[24] Jayaprakasam A, Darvay A, Osborne G, McGibbon D. Comparison of assessment of severity and quality of life in cutaneous disease. Clinical and Experimental Dermatology. 2002;**27**:306-308

[25] Aghaei S, Saki N, Daneshmand E, Kardeh B. Prevalence of psychological disorders in patients with alopecia areata in comparison with normal subjects. ISRN Dermatology. 2014;**2014**:304370. DOI: 10.1155/2014/304370

[26] Pawaskar MD, Parikh P, Markowski T, et al. Melasma and its impact on health-related quality of life in Hispanic women. Journal of Dermatological Treatment. 2007;**18**:5-9

Chapter 2

Melasma: A Review about Pathophysiology and Treatment

Marisa Gonzaga da Cunha and Ana Paula da Silva Urzedo

Abstract

Melasma is a very common disease that is manifested by increased skin pigmentation mostly in the face but also in the décolleté, neck, and arms. It is presented as irregular, light to dark brown spots, placed on the forehead. Cheek bones, mandible, and supralabial region. It usually affects women in higher phototypes (III–V), more commonly at a rate of nine women: one man. Melasma is a multifactorial disease, and we know that some conditions, such as pregnancy, contraceptives, thyroid diseases, hormone replacement, and solar exposure, could be a trigger to develop this illness. Despite not being a serious condition, melasma causes discomfort for those who have it, and it could compromise the patient's quality of life. The goal of this chapter is to understand the pathogenic mechanism of melasma as well as revise the treatments of this disorder.

Keywords: melasma, melasma treatments, melasma oral treatments, laser, pulsed light intense, peelings and melasma, hormones and melasma

1. Introduction

Melasma is a condition that affects millions of individuals around the world, most often women than men, in the proportion of 9:1. Although it is not a serious disease, it has a very important psychological impact on people who suffer from this condition.

It is known to affect people with higher phototypes; it is related to exposure to UV radiation and visible light, as well as thyroid disorders, and the use of contraceptives, hormone replacement, and drugs for epilepsy [1, 2].

2. Methodology

The authors made research on the platform PubMed with the terms: "melasma," "melasma and treatment," melasma and pathophysiology," "melasma and new treatments," "melasma and oral treatments," and "melasma and laser."

More than 10,660 papers were found. The papers included in this chapter have been published in the last 5 years.

3. Objective

The objective of this chapter is to review the pathophysiology of Melasma and discuss both current treatments and the ones about to come.

4. Etiopathogenesis

For a better understanding of pigmentation disorders, it is important to understand the biology of melanocytes, which are neural crest-derived cells. During embryogenesis, melanocytes' precursor's cells, called melanoblasts, migrate along the dorsolateral pathway to reach the epidermis and hair follicles.

Causes for the increase in the production of melanin:

1. Expression of proopiomelanocortin (POMC) and its derivatives by cells within the skin;

2. Number of melanocortin-1 receptors (MC1-R) on melanocytes;

3. Release of diacylglycerol (DAG) from the plasma membrane that activates protein kinase C;

4. Induction of SOS reaction for UVR-induced cell damage;

5. Production of nitric oxide (NO) that activates the cGMP pathway;

6. Production of cytokines and growth factors by keratinocytes [3].

Five main etiopathogenic mechanisms have been detected in melasma:

1. Inappropriate activation of melanocytes;

2. Aggregation of melanin and melanosomes in the dermis and epidermis;

3. Increased number of mast cells and solar elastosis;

4. Basement membrane changes;

5. Increased vascularization.

4.1 Inappropriate activation of melanocytes

The melanocytes are more active in the area of the melasma, and when exposed to UV radiation or visible light, they increase the production of melanin through organelles called melanosomes.

Melanin synthesis is closely related to the enzyme tyrosinase, which, in addition to several other enzymatic processes, will convert tyrosine into eumelanin. After this conversion, melanin will be distributed to the keratinocytes. Keratinocytes, fibroblasts, and other cells of the immune system will secrete paracrine factors related to either inflammatory stimuli or sunlight.

Extracellular matrix (ECM) glycoproteins in peripheral cutaneous nerves can also be affected by melanogenesis. These mechanisms increase the amount of melanin in keratinocytes in the epidermis and macrophages in the dermis.

The receptor for tyrosine kinase (c-KIT) is able to place phosphate groups on the tyrosine residues of other proteins, as well as activate autophosphorylation. The KIT binding membrane (m-KIT) and its soluble form (s-KIT) have demonstrated antagonistic mechanisms *in vivo* and *in vitro*. The binding of stem cell factors (SCF) to m-KIT induces melanogenesis, while the s-KIT production suppresses melanogenesis in human melanocyte culture.

UVB radiation increases SCF and m-KIT levels and decreases s-KIT expression levels, resulting in increased melanogenesis. The increase in SCF levels in the dermis together with the increase in c-KIT in the epidermis of patients with melasma is partially mediated through cell-cell interactions between melanocytes and fibroblasts.

Fibroblasts secrete Wnt signaling modulators, which stimulate both melanogenesis and melanosome transfer. The Wnt/β-catenin pathway includes a large family of proteins with different cellular functions, such as melanoblast migration, proliferation, and pigmentation induction. Wnt1 is a beaded transmembrane receptor binding, which promotes the accumulation and stabilization of β-catenin. When incubated in cell culture, melasma fibroblasts also enhance melanogenesis, with overexpression of nerve-derived growth factor.

Another implicated factor is the UV radiation that induces cyclooxygenase (COX-2). COX-2 knock-down in melanocytes results in decreased expression of tyrosinase, protein-1 (TRP-1), TRP-2, glycoprotein 100, and MITF. Besides, COX-2 siRNA-transfected melanocytes show a reduction of alpha MSH.

Despite the whole face being exposed to the sun, it can be observed that only some areas, mainly the ones rich in sebaceous glands, will be affected by melasma. This may be due to the fact that these appendages have the ability to synthesize vitamin D and secrete various cytokines and growth factors. Sebocytes are controlled by alpha-MSH, which suggests a connection between these cells and melanocytes. Moreover, skin surface lipids undergo oxidation by UVR, which can activate melanin synthesis in melanocyte culture.

There is also a marked increase in superoxide dismutase activity, as well as a significant reduction in glutathione levels in melasma patients, leading to the belief that these people suffer from increased oxidative stress [4, 5].

4.2 Aggregation of melanin and melanosomes in the dermis and epidermis

Biopsies of areas affected by melasma demonstrate melanin increase in both epidermis and dermis when compared to perilesional skin.

Rupture of the basement membrane causes melanocytes to descend into the dermis as free melanocytes (melanocyte effusion). On electron microscopy, it can be seen that melanocytes in the area with melasma have more dendrites than those in normal skin. They also have more mitochondria, golgi complex, rough endoplasmic reticulum, and ribosomes in their cytoplasm [4].

4.3 Increased number of mast cells and solar elastosis

Solar elastosis is the abnormal accumulation of elastic tissue in a dermis that is chronically exposed to the sun, and this occurs in 83–93% of patients with melasma.

Mast cells are most prominent in the elastotic areas of the skin affected by melasma. In the development of solar elastosis, mast cells have been shown to induce fibroblasts to produce elastin, either directly or indirectly through other cells or cytokines. Mast cells are capable of inducing vascular proliferation by various angiogenic factors, such as VEGF, basic fibroblast growth factor (bFGF-2), and transforming growth factor beta (TGF-β).

Mast cell tryptase and granzyme B are involved in basement membrane degradation after UV irradiation. Mast cells are involved with solar elastosis, vasodilation, and basement membrane rupture, which can be seen in histology [4].

4.4 Basement membrane changes

The rupture of the basement membrane (BM) is described in several studies. Vacuolar degeneration of basement cells and vacuolar degeneration of the basement membrane and subbasement membrane region have been described.

Chronic exposure to UV radiation results in increased levels of matrix metalloproteinase 2 (MMP2), which degrades collagens IV and VI, leading to basement membrane rupture. This allows melanocytes to descend through the dermis, which is known as pendant melanocytes, and they can contribute to pigmentation both during their migration into the dermis and after trauma or treatment.

BM damage, due to aging, environment, and iatrogenic factors, could facilitate the migration of active melanocytes and melanin to the dermis, leading to the accumulation of free melanin or melanophages, thus explaining the persistent hyperpigmentation in melasma.

BM degradation is also mediated by mast cells as seen above. The degradation of these cells releases tryptase that can activate MMPs and cause direct damage to extracellular matrix proteins.

Granzyme B, a serine protease expressed by a variety of immune and nonimmune cells (including mast cells), accumulates in the extracellular space during chronic inflammation and cleavage of various extracellular matrix proteins, possibly leading to the ECM degradation after UV irradiation.

Melasma presents an accumulation of photodamaged fibroblasts, which leads us to believe that the aging caused by UV radiation may be involved in the genesis of this disease.

BM degradation may facilitate the transfer of multiple growth factors between dermis and epidermis, which could lead to persistent hyperpigmentation [4].

4.5 Increased vascularization

A pronounced increase in vascularity is seen in melasma, and this can also be observed in various inflammatory conditions, including the response to UV radiation.

Vascular endothelial growth factor (VEGF) is increased in the vessels in areas affected by melasma. Normal human melanocytes express VEGF receptors in vitro. Some of these receptors are functional, suggesting that VEGF plays a role in melanocyte behavior in the skin.

VEGF binds to specific receptors, which are also found on endothelial cells that have been shown to stimulate pigmentation through the production of endothelin 1. Endothelin 1 is released by the endothelium of microvessels inducing melanogenesis, characterized by MIFT phosphorylation and increased tyrosinase levels. VEGF also influences melanocytes by stimulating the release of arachidonic acid and the subsequent activation of phospholipase A. The increased production of melanin may result from metabolites that are secreted in the arachidonic acid pathway. VEGF may also partially affect pigmentation through positive regulation of the expression of protease-activated receptors (PAR-2), especially in melasma patients with prominent telangiectatic erythema.

Sex hormones alone, mainly estrogen, are not capable of inducing melasma pigmentation, but they act synergistically with UVB radiation. However, estrogen can perpetuate hyperpigmentation by increasing vascularity, which, in turn, stimulates endothelin 1 secretion. As the sensitivity of cells to sex hormones is an individual factor, this could probably explain the variability in susceptibility to developing the disease [2, 4].

4.6 The role of visible light in melasma

A follow-up study by Regazzetti *et al.* was performed on normal human melanocytes (NHMs) in order to understand the mechanisms of blue-light-induced hyperpigmentation. Blue light has been shown to stimulate melanogenesis by acting on the microphthalmia-associated transcription factor (MITF), the master pigmentation gene.

Photons are absorbed and converted into a cellular response through a class of G-protein-coupled receptors called opsins, which are light-activated. Traditionally, opsins are well known for their role in the photoreception of the eye. However, recent studies have shown that rhodopsin (OPN2), cone opsins (OPN1-SW), encephalopsin/opsin-3 (OPN3), and neuropsin (OPN5) are expressed both in melanocytes and keratinocytes. Notably, OPN2 and OPN3 were significantly more abundant than other opsins. In Regazzetti's study, after irradiating normal human melanocytes with blue light, OPN3 was the only significantly expressed opsin. To investigate whether OPN3 could mediate the effects of blue light melanogenesis, OPN3 was knocked down using small interfering RNA (siRNA). In NHMs with siRNA directed against OPN3, blue light irradiation no longer had an effect on MITF phosphorylation [6].

5. Treatment

As melasma has a lot of pathways to induce melanogenesis, the treatment must include many topical and systemic drugs. Antioxidants and photo protectors, as well as lightning, laser, peeling, and other procedures are usually indicated.

In the paragraph below, we will discuss the indicated treatments and their mechanisms of action (**Tables 1** and **2**).

Treating melasma is a challenge, and it is known that the treatment must address the various mechanisms of hyperpigmentation of this condition.

The most frequently cited depigmenting topical agent in literature is still hydroquinone. It works by inhibiting the conversion of 1–3,4-dihydroxyphenylalanine into melanin by competitive inhibition of tyrosinase. Although the risk seems to be only theoretical, there might be side effects, such as exogenous ochronosis, permanent depigmentation, and potential carcinogenic risk.

Up to now, other depigmenting agents considered safer to date are 4-n-butylresorcinol, niacinamide, ascorbic acid, resveratrol, azelaic acid, and kojic acid. However, depigmenting agents alone are not able to improve the photoaging issue closely related to melasma. Therefore, antiaging agents should be associated in order to try

Active	Mechanism of action	Drug concentration
Hydroquinone	Tyrosinase inhibitor	2–4%
4-N-butyl resorcinol	Tyrosinase inhibitor	2–4%
Niacinamide	Reduction of melanosome transfer anti-inflammatory antiaging	5–10%
Ascorbic acid	Antioxidant Tyrosinase inhibitor photoprotective effects	5–25%
Azelaic acid	Antiaging effect antiaging	10–20%
Kojic acid	Tyrosinase inhibitor trapping free radicals	1–4%
Triple combination Hydroquinone tretinoin, fluocinolone acetonide	Depigment effect Tyrosinase inhibitor Anti-inflammatory effect	4%, 0,05% 0,01%
Arbutin	Tyrosinase inhibitor	1–3%
N-acetyl-4 s cysteamine phenol (NCAP4%)	Antioxidant effects	5%
Resveratrol	Melanogenesis inhibitor Tyrosinase inhibitor	1%

Table 1.
Mainly topical treatments for melasma.

Korean red ginseng powder	Korean red ginseng powder shows good tolerability and beneficial effects for melasma
Polypodium leucotomos	Oral PLE is not significantly better than placebo as an adjunct to topical sunscreen for melasma oral polypodium leucotomos extract appears to be a safe and effective adjunctive treatment in combination with topical hydroquinone and sunscreen for melasma
Pycnogenol/grape seed extract	Pycnogenol 75 mg is therapeutically effective and safe in patients suffering from melasma Grape seed extract is safe and useful for improving chloasma
Vitamin E	Vitamin C + E combination treatment has significantly better results than vitamin C alone for chloasma Oral procyanidin + vitamins A, C, and E are safe and effective for epidermal melasma.
Refs. [7–10].	

Table 2.
Oral treatments for melasma.

and correct the photodamage, as this may be related to the frequent recurrences of this condition.

The triple combination containing hydroquinone (HQ) 4%, 0.05% tretinoin, and 0.01% fluocinolone acetonide is the only FDA-approved drug that contains HQ for the treatment of melasma. Tretinoin has depigmenting and antiaging effects. Steroids inhibit the secretion of both ET-1 and granulocyte-macrophage colony-stimulating factor (GM-CSF), acting against the inflammation present in melasma, which is related to photodamage and melanogenesis. Azelaic acid is an anti-inflammatory agent with depigmenting properties that have been reported to reverse the aging of human fibroblasts after PUVA induction. It also inhibits the secretion of MMP-1 and growth factors, such as the hepatocyte growth factor (HGF) and the

SCF, through the activation of the peroxisome proliferator-activated gamma receptor (PPARy).

Wnt antagonists, including cardamonin and FTY720 (fingolimod), have been shown to suppress melanogenesis in vitro. A recent study has demonstrated that andropholide inhibits tyrosinase activity and melanin production via the Beta-catenin degradation into B16F10 in the UVB-induced melanoma cells in guinea pigs [6].

5.1 New topical agents that target hyperactive melanocytes

Linoleic acid: has selectivity for tyrosinase in hyperactive melanocytes and decreases UVB-induced hyperpigmentation.

Ascorbic acid: decreases dopaquinone oxidation into DHICA dihydrxyindole-2-carboxylic acid), lowers tyrosinase activity, reduces dermal damage, promotes collagen synthesis, and has both antioxidant and photoprotective effects, thus reducing pigmentation.

N-acetyl-4S cysteamine phenol (NCAP4%): less irritating and more stable than hydroquinone, is a tyrosinase inhibitor in hyperactive melanocytes, interfering with the thiol system, decreasing intracellular glutathione, and favoring pheomelanin synthesis [11].

5.2 New agents targeting melanogenesis

Aloesin: aloe vera extract that inhibits the conversion of tyrosinase into DOPA and of DOPA to dopachrome.

Rucinol (4-n-butylresorcinol): a phenolic derivative that inhibits tyrosinase and TYRP-1.

Flavonoids: benzopyrene derivatives, which are competitive inhibitors of tyrosinase with anti-inflammatory effects and antioxidant properties. Hesperidin: a flavonoid that protects against free radical-induced damage caused by UVR.

Epigallocatechin gallate: a phenolic compound, extracted from green tea, which inhibits melanogenesis and has a significant anti-inflammatory, antioxidant and anti-cancer effect.

Ellagic acid: a polyphenol derived from green tea, strawberries, and pomegranate that can inhibit tyrosinase and melanocytic proliferation.

Gentisic acid: a compound extracted from the gentile roots that inhibit melanin synthesis.

Hydroxycoumarin: occurs naturally in lactones that inhibit tyrosinase due to their antioxidant action. Umbelliferone (7-hydroxycoumarin) has anti-inflammatory action.

Cinnamic acid: derived from ginseng, inhibits tyrosinase and is more potent than hydroquinone.

Antisense oligonucleotides: act as a bleaching agent by downregulating the production of enzymes that involve melanogenesis and decrease the activity of DOPA oxidase [11].

5.3 Agents against reactive oxygen species (ROS) and inflammation

Liquorice extract: derived from the root of *Glycyrrhiza glabra*, inhibits melanin synthesis and disperses melanin, in addition to decreasing ROS production. It has anti-inflammatory effects and decreases UVB-induced hyperpigmentation in guinea pigs after 3 weeks of use.

Acidified amino acid peels: peels with a pH close to the skin's pH have antioxidant and tyrosinase inhibitory effects.

Orchid extract: strong antioxidant activity. It has proven to be as effective as vitamin C in a study with 48 melasma patients.

Coffeeberry extract: has antioxidant properties and reduces hyperpigmentation as well as photodamage.

Mulberry extract: derived from the *Morus alba*, its extract is a free radical chelator and a tyrosinase inhibitor.

Pycnogenol (oral): derived from the bark of *Pinus pinaster*, it presents antioxidant and anti-inflammatory activity.

Polypodium leucotomos (oral): this extract works by inhibiting UVR-induced ROS, including superoxide anions.

Alpha tocopherol: strong anti-inflammatory and marked antioxidant activity.

Proanthocyanidin (oral): grape seed extract with antioxidant action. A study conducted on women submitted to a 6-month treatment has shown whitening in 10 out of 12 women [11].

5.4 Melanosomal transfer: Protease-activated receptor2

Niacinamide or vitamin B3: active amide of niacin, interferes with melanosome transfer to the surrounding keratinocytes by inhibiting PAR-2.

Liquiritin: leads to a skin-lightening effect through dispersion of melanin.

Soymilk, soybean (topical): the serine protease inhibitors, such as soy trypsin inhibitor (STI) and Bowman-Birk inhibitor (BBI), found in soybeans have been shown to inhibit melanosome phagocytosis by keratinocytes via the inhibition of PAR-2. Newer agents that target the defective barrier, such as soy topically applied and active soy moisturizers containing nondenatured serine protease inhibitors (STI and BBI), can decrease UVB-induced pigmentation by restoring the skin barrier [11].

5.5 Agents targeting the vascular component

The systemic tranexamic acid (TXA) is an anti-fibrinolytic agent, which has been shown to be an inhibitor of both UV-radiation-induced melanogenesis and neovascularization, by blocking the plasminogen activator and plasmin activity. Oral administration is at a dose of 250 mg from 2 to 3 times a day for 2 to 3 months, with a significant decrease in both melanin and erythema indexes in the skin with melanin lesions. Histology demonstrates a decrease in pigment, number of vessels, and mast cells. There is a decrease in ET-1 expression. Despite being well tolerated, we must be aware that this drug has, in theory, thrombogenic potential. TXA can also be injected in intradermotherapy associated with lasers and microneedling, but there are not enough studies and the results are still limited [11].

5.6 Agents that target mast cells

5.6.1 Tranexamic acid

Zinc: reduces mast cell secretion and has an antioxidant effect [11].

5.7 Agents with hormonal targets

Flutamide is an antiandrogenic agent that can influence alpha-melanocyte-stimulating hormone and cyclic adenosine monophosphate, which are key regulators of melanogenesis [11].

5.8 Newer agents with unique mechanisms: Potential targets of the future

Curcumin (topical) is a bioactive compound extracted from the rhizome of *Curcuma longa* and its use is well-established in traditional Chinese medicine for the treatment of various skin diseases. It inhibits UVB-induced production of ROS and the expression of matrix metalloproteinase in vitro by blocking the activation of the UVB-induced mitogen-activated protein kinase, the nuclear factor-κB, and the AP-1 transcription factor signal pathway. Curcumin gel has been useful in the repair of photodamaged skin as well as for the associated pigmentary changes and solar elastosis. In view of its anti-inflammatory, free radical scavenging, and UV-protective activities, curcumin may serve as a new skin-lightening agent in the future, both in topical and oral preparations.

Lignin peroxidase (LP, topical use) is an enzyme derived from the fungus Phanerochaete chrysosporium. Since lignin is structurally similar to melanin, lignin-degrading enzymes can be utilized to decolorize melanin. Lignin peroxidase is marketed as a formulation containing the active enzymatic component and its activator (hydrogen peroxide), causing the destruction of eumelanin.

Treatments with technologies, such as intense pulsed light (IPL), fractional laser, 1550 nm nonablative laser, Q-Switched neodynium-doped yttrium aluminum garnet laser (QSNYL), pulsed dye laser (PDL), and copper-bromide laser, have shown positive results. Laser toning using collimated, low fluence, 1064 nm QSNYL removes melanosomes and damages the dendrites of melanocytes without destroying the entire melanocyte ("subcellular selective photothermolysis"). Nevertheless, the accumulation of energy from several sessions can cause depigmented mottling lesions similar to scars, which makes melanogenesis difficult [11, 12].

Newer sunscreens: visible light (VL) and infrared light (IR) have been shown to play an important role in hyperpigmentation, especially in the darker skin types (III, IV, or V). VL may induce the production of ROS, leading to DNA damage. IR light provokes the activation of the endothelin receptor B and the mitogen-activated protein kinase, which facilitates melanogenesis. Sunscreens containing iron-oxide are effective against hyperpigmentation induced by VL.

Other new UV-VL sunscreens that allow absorption of the radiation in the VL spectrum and systemic antioxidants, such as vitamin A, C, and E, carotenoids, and beta-carotene, may provide additive protection. Nonorganic and organic filters that absorb or reflect IR are currently available. Also, topical antioxidants may be able to offer some protection against IR-related damage. However, their clinical efficacy remains to be determined.

6. Discussion

Melasma is a multifactorial disease and until now there is not a universal treatment to solve it. At the moment, the first choice to treat melasma is the triple association of tretinoin, hydroquinone, and fluocinolone acetonide associated with a broad-spectrum pigmented sunscreen, but this treatment presents some side effects, such as exogenous ochronosis and depigmentation, in confetti when used for a long time. Despite all the knowledge about the pathophysiology of melasma, we do not have the cure for the disease. There are many new drugs with different targets to control the pigmentation, but, unfortunately, there is often resurgence of melasma. The discovery of the influence of the vessels in the pathogenesis of melasma was very important, and there are some papers about the use of oral tranexamic acid with encouraging results, but these treatment regimens must be reserved for refractory cases.

Concerning peeling, laser, and other technologies, some publications show good results, but there is not a big study with a long follow-up period to confirm efficacy. It is very important to bear in mind that melasma is a chronic disease and these treatments, which are very expensive for the patients, could sometimes generate false expectations.

7. Conclusion

Melasma is a very common disease that is a challenge to manage. More research about de pathogenesis of the disease is necessary, leading to the development of new drugs and therapies to control it.

To sum up, the most interesting approach to treat the disease involves a rotation of treatments and removing the causes that worsen the condition, as well as teaching the patient to make up and camouflage the lesions.

8. Key points in this chapter

1. Melasma is a multifactorial disease.

2. Sunscreen with pigment has a very important role in the treatment.

3. Topical treatment with different targets in the pathophysiology of melasma could control the disease.

4. Laser, peelings, and micro-needling could be an interesting adjuvant treatment.

Author details

Marisa Gonzaga da Cunha[1] and Ana Paula da Silva Urzedo[2]*

1 Cosmiatry Department, Faculdade de Medicina do ABC Department of Dermatology, SP, Brazil

2 Cosmiatry Clinic, Faculdade de Medicina do ABC Department of Dermatology, Brazil

*Address all correspondence to: apurzedo.71@gmail.com

References

[1] Kheradmand M, Afshari M, Damiani G, Abediankenari S, et al. Melasma and thyroid disorders: A systematic review and meta-analysis. International Journal of Dermatology. 2019;**58**(11):1231-1238

[2] Rajanala S, Maymone MBC, Vashi NA. Melasma pathogenesis: A review of the latest research, pathological findings, and investigational therapies. Dermatology Online Journal. 2019;**25**(10):1-6

[3] Kwon SH, Na JI, Choi JY, Park KC. Melasma: Updates and perspectives. Experimental Dermatology. 2019;**28**(6):704-708

[4] Artzi O, Horovitz T, Bar-Ilan E, Shehadeh W, et al. The pathogenesis of melasma and implications for treatment. Journal of Cosmetic Dermatology. 2021;**20**(11):3432-3445

[5] Espósito ACC, Brianezi G, de Souza NP, Miot LDB, et al. Exploratory study of epidermis, basement membrane zone, upper dermis alterations and Wnt pathway activation in Melasma compared to adjacent and Retroauricular skin. Annals of Dermatology. 2020;**32**(2):101-108

[6] Narla S, Kohli I, Hamzavi IH, Lim HW. Visible light in photodermatology. Photochemical & Photobiological Sciences. 2020;**19**(1):99-104

[7] Babbush KM, Babbush RA, Khachemoune A. Treatment of melasma: A review of less commonly used antioxidants. International Journal of Dermatology. 2021;**60**(2):166-173

[8] Boo YC. Arbutin as a skin depigmenting agent with Antimelanogenic and antioxidant properties. Antioxidants (Basel). 2021;**10**(7):2-22

[9] Farris P, Zeichner J, Berson D. Efficacy and tolerability of a skin brightening/anti-aging cosmeceutical containing retinol 0.5%, Niacinamide, hexylresorcinol, and resveratrol. Journal of Drugs in Dermatology. 2016;**15**(7):863-868

[10] Kwon SH, Yang JH, Shin JW, Park KC, et al. Efficacy of liposome-encapsulated 4-n-butylresorcinol and resveratrol cream in the treatment of melasma. Journal of Cosmetic Dermatology. 2020;**19**(4):891-895

[11] Sarkar R, Bansal A, Ailawadi P. Future therapies in melasma: What lies ahead? Indian Journal of Dermatology, Venereology and Leprology. 2020;**86**(1):8-17

[12] Lai D, Zhou S, Cheng S, Liu H, et al. Laser therapy in the treatment of melasma: A systematic review and meta-analysis. Lasers in Medical Science. 2022;**37**(4):2099-2110

Section 2

Hypopigmentation Disorders

Chapter 3

Vitiligo: Pathogenesis, Clinical Features, and Treatment

Emine Müge Acar

Abstract

Vitiligo is a depigmenting skin disorder of unknown etiology, which presents with nonscaly, chalky-white macules. Selective loss of melanocytes is the characteristic feature of vitiligo. Of the many theories proposed for melanocyte loss, convergence theory, which suggests that the combination of biochemical, environmental, and immunological factors play a role in the pathophysiology of vitiligo, is currently the most accepted theory. Treatment options include topical and systemic immunosuppressants, phototherapy, and surgical techniques. The subtype, extent, distribution, and activity of disease are the determining factors for treatment choice. In this chapter, the pathogenesis, clinical features of vitiligo, and treatment options are discussed.

Keywords: vitiligo, pathogenesis, clinical features, treatment

1. Introduction

Vitiligo is a pigmentation disorder characterized by depigmented macules and patches on the skin. The prevalence of vitiligo ranges from 0.4 to 2.0% worldwide. Vitiligo has no predilection for age, gender, racial background, or skin types [1, 2]. The peak period of onset is between 10–30 years, although it can develop at any age [3–6].

Vitiligo is classified as an autoimmune disease having a genetic basis and an association with environmental factors, including chemical triggers, skin injury, sunburn, and virus infection. Vitiligo is considered to develop as a result of metabolic, oxidative stress, and cell detachment abnormalities [7, 8].

Vitiligo is classified into two major forms: nonsegmental vitiligo (NSV) and segmental vitiligo (SV) [2]. Nonsegmental vitiligo includes acrofacial, mucosal, generalized, universal, mixed, and rare variants. Generalized vitiligo is the most common subtype which often involves the face and acral regions [9].

Vitiligo is a psychologically devastating skin disease, and it is associated with depression, stress, fear, shame, insecurity, sadness, and low self-esteem, which could lead to social isolation or even suicidal ideation [10–13].

Therefore, vitiligo has considerable psychological and social effects on daily life [3].

IntechOpen

2. Etiology and pathogenesis

Vitiligo is characterized by the destruction of melanocytes, which leads to pigment loss in the affected areas. The pathogenesis of vitiligo has not yet been fully elucidated. Various theories, including autoimmune theory, adhesion defect theory, biochemical and neural theory, viral theory, intrinsic theory, zinc-α2-glycoprotein deficiency hypothesis and biochemical, and molecular and cellular alterations accounting for the loss of functioning melanocytes in vitiligo have been proposed [14]. Familial aggregation of vitiligo supports the genetic basis of the disease. HLA-associated genes, including HLA-A2, HLA-DR4, and HLA-DR7 alleles [15–17] and non-HLA genes, including DDR1, XBP1, NLRP1, PTPN22, and COMT [18] have been linked to vitiligo susceptibility.

2.1 Autoimmune theory

The autoimmune theory of vitiligo proposes that autoimmune effector mechanisms are involved in melanocyte destruction. The association of vitiligo with several autoimmune diseases, including autoimmune thyroid diseases, alopecia areata, halo nevi, and Addison's disease supports the autoimmune basis of vitiligo [19–23]. Several circulating autoantibodies having a specificity for pigment cells have been detected in sera of vitiligo patients. Antimelanocyte antibodies, especially against tyrosinase one and two (TRP-1 and TRP-2) are found in high levels in about 10% of patients [24–27]. Although the role of antimelanocyte antibodies in vitiligo is still not well known. These autoantibodies are currently considered to develop as a consequence of secondary humoral response to melanocyte destruction [28]. Studies revealing CD4+ and CD8+ lymphocytes in the dermal-epidermal junction of areas of skin near a vitiligo lesion suggest the activation of cell-mediated immunity in vitiligo [29, 30]. Cytotoxic CD8+ T cells, which recognize melanocyte-specific antigens, such as tyrosinase, Melan-A/MART-1, gp100, TRP-1, and TRP-2, have been shown to exert anti-melanocytic cytotoxic activity *in vitro* [31, 32]. Elevation of tumor necrosis factor-α (TNF-α), interferon-γ (IFN γ), and IL-10 and IL-17 also have been demonstrated in the blood and tissues of vitiligo patients [33, 34].

2.2 Adhesion defect theory

"Melanocytorrhagy" theory, proposed by Gauthier et al. in 2003 suggests that the major predisposing factor for the development of vitiligo is the primary defective adhesion in the epidermis due to the defective synthesis of extracellular matrix components by keratinocytes and the impaired formation of the basement membrane [35, 36]. This theory argues that chronic detachment and transepidermal loss of melanocytes caused by trauma underlies vitiligo pathogenesis, which is also supported by koebnerization, seen in vitiligo lesions. Overexpression of tenascin in vitiligo patients may play a role in decreasing melanocyte adhesion [37]. Autoantigens released during melanocytorrhagy are hypothesized to cause autoimmune activation provoked by dendritic cells or memory T cells [35, 36].

2.3 Biochemical theory

The biochemical hypothesis argues that biochemical abnormalities of melanocytes and keratinocytes leading to aberrant melanization are involved in vitiligo pathogenesis. Oxidative stress is implicated in the destruction of melanocytes [37–40]. Defective free radical defense, excessive quantities of hydrogen peroxide (H_2O_2), and the accumulation of toxic intermediate metabolites of melanin synthesis are suggested to play a role in this process [41]. Danger signals named damage-associated molecular patterns (DAMPs), including reactive oxygen species (ROS) and iHSP70, are released from stressed melanocytes [42]. Reactive oxygen species (ROS) lead to the imbalance of prooxidant and antioxidant systems in favor of the prooxidant system. Elevation of oxidative stress markers (superoxide dismutase, malondialdehyde, and ROS) and a reduction of antioxidative enzymes (catalase, glutathione peroxidase, glutathione reductase, thioredoxin reductase, thioredoxin, and superoxide dismutases), and the repair enzymes result with the increased sensitivity of melanocytes to external prooxidant stimuli [37–39]. Defective function of mitochondria, such as alterations in the mitochondrial transmembrane potential and in the electron transport chain, is also suggested to play a role in the pathophysiology of vitiligo [37, 43, 44].

Oxidative stress also affects the recycling of tetrahydrobiopterin, which acts as an essential cofactor in the synthesis of L-tyrosine from L-phenylalanine in tyrosinase synthesis [14]. Tyrosinase is a key enzyme in the formation of melanin [45]. Oxidative stress modifies the active site of dihydropteridin reductase, which plays a role in the recycling process of 6-tetrahydrobiopterin [39]. As a result, the production of hydrogen peroxide increases, and catalase levels decrease, contributing to melanocyte death [46, 47].

2.4 Neural theory

The "neural theory," which was proposed by Lerner's suggests that dysfunction of the sympathetic nervous system (SNS) affects the melanin production and causes depigmentation [48]. The cutaneous blood flow was found approximately three times higher on the segmental vitiligo lesions *than on* normal skin with iontophoresis and laser Doppler flowmetry [49]. Elevated levels of nerve growth factor (NGF), and correlation of HVA and VMA levels with disease activity have been reported in vitiligo patients [50]. Mental stress can also trigger the secretion of catecholamines by stimulating the hypothalamic-pituitary-adrenal axis [51, 52]. Catecholamine discharge induced by stressors leads to vasoconstriction, hypoxia, and overproduction of oxygen radicals that cause melanocyte destruction [51, 52].

2.5 Viral theory

Chronic hepatitis C virus (HCV) infection and autoimmune hepatitis are found strongly associated with vitiligo [53]. A low hepatitis B virus (HBV) seropositivity in vitiligo patients has been reported [54]. Previous or concurrent cytomegalovirus (CMV) infections may play a role in vitiligo onset or deterioration of the disease [55]. Epstein-Barr virus, hepatitis E virus, and the human immunodeficiency virus (HIV) also have been implicated in vitiligo pathogenesis [55–59].

2.6 Zinc-α2-Glycoprotein deficiency hypothesis

The hypothesis that a probable association may exist between Zinc-α2-Glycoprotein (ZAG) deficiency and vitiligo was proposed by Bagherani et al. and Yaghoobi et al. [60, 61]. The ZAG is a 41000 Da adipokine involved in lipolysis, regulation of metabolism, cell proliferation and differentiation, cell adhesion, and immunoregulation [62, 63]. Zinc-α2-glycoprotein (ZAG) is secreted from keratinocytes and influences melanocyte proliferation, dendricity, and melanin synthesis [64, 65]. Decreased levels of ZAG detected in vitiligo patients support this theory [66].

2.7 Intrinsic theory

The intrinsic theory implies that an intrinsic defect in melanocytes may be the causal factor for melanocyte death. The abnormal rough endoplasmic reticulum, deficiency of melanocyte growth factors, such as basic fibroblast growth factor (bFGF) and decrease in the number of melanocytes, expressing the c-kit receptor in lesional skin may play a role in melanocyte damage [67, 68].

2.8 Apoptosis and accelerated cell senescence

Melanocytes from non-lesional skin of vitiligo patients show some cytologic changes, including cytoplasm vacuolization, DNA marginalization in the nucleus, loss of dendrites, and detachment [67, 69, 70]. In addition, degeneration of basal and suprabasal epidermal cells in the depigmented and normally pigmented skin due to swelling of the membrane-bound organelles, formation of vacuoles, and cytoplasm condensation are among the apoptotic changes [71]. The lower expression levels of the antiapoptotic Bcl-2, FLIP proteins in vitiliginous skin, high levels of the proapoptotic bax, p53 proteins, and of the active forms of caspase-3, 8, and 9 contribute to the apoptotic process in vitiligo [72, 73]. Modification of proliferation and senescence marker expressions (p16, p53, and p21) is another finding reported in vitiligo lesions when compared to keratinocytes from noninvolved skin [73].

2.9 Integrated theory (Convergence theory)

Convergence theory argues that vitiligo may be a syndrome with a multi-factorial etiology rather than a single entity. Since the pathophysiology of vitiligo cannot be sufficiently explained by immune or nonimmune mechanisms, this theory suggesting that the combination of biochemical, environmental, and immunological factors play a role in the pathophysiology of vitiligo is currently the most accepted theory [74].

3. Clinic

The clinical manifestation of vitiligo is chalk-white or milk-white patches with various sizes ranging from a few millimeters to several centimeters. The lesions are generally asymptomatic itching/burning sensation may rarely occur in vitiligo onset [75]. Vitiligo has a chronic, unpredictable course with remissions and exacerbations. The disease is often progressive; spontaneous repigmentation occurs in 10–20% of patients [61].

The term non-segmental vitiligo (NSV) refers to all forms of vitiligo that are not classified as segmental vitiligo (acrofacial, mucosal, generalized, universal, mixed, and rare variants). Segmental vitiligo tends to have an earlier age of onset than NSV [76].

3.1 Non-segmental vitiligo subsets (NSV)

3.1.1 Acrofacial

Acrofacial vitiligo clinically presents as depigmented macules localized on the face, head, and distal extremities. The perioral and periocular regions are preferably involved. Vitiligo lesions in the genital areas are also classified in this group. Progression to generalized or universal vitiligo can be seen during the disease course.

3.1.2 Generalized common vitiligo

Generalized vitiligo is characterized by bilateral, often symmetrical, depigmented macules or patches involving multiple parts of the body. Hands, fingers, and face are the most frequent sites involved at the onset. The areas exposed to pressure, friction, and trauma are often affected [9].

3.1.3 Vitiligo universalis

Vitiligo universalis is the most widespread form of vitiligo that is characterized by the involvement of 80–90% of the body surface. It is generally preceded by generalized vitiligo [7].

3.1.4 Mixed vitiligo

Mixed vitiligo is the concomitant existence of segmental and non-segmental vitiligo. Non-segmental vitiligo is generally preceded by segmental form. The clinical features are: (1) the absence of depigmented areas in a segmental distribution at birth and in the first year of life and exclusion of nevus depigmentosus by Wood lamp examination; (2) NSV development following SV after a period of at least 6 months; (3) SV involving at least 20% of the dermatomal segment or following a definite Blaschko linear distribution; (4) different treatment responses to conventional narrow band ultraviolet B (NB-UVB) between SV (poor response) and NSV (good response). The presence of leukotrichia and halo nevi at onset in patients with SV may be risk factors for developing mixed vitiligo [77].

3.1.5 Mucosal vitiligo

Oral and/or genital mucosae are typically involved. Mucosal vitiligo may be an isolated condition or may occur in the course of generalized vitiligo.

3.1.6 Rare forms

Vitiligo punctata is characterized by 1- to 1.5-mm sized, sharply demarcated depigmented, and punctiform macules affecting any area of the body [78].

Hypochromic vitiligo or vitiligo minor refers to a partial defect in pigmentation resulting from hypopigmented macules. A seborrheic distribution on the face and neck is seen. Hypochromic vitiligo exclusively affects dark-skinned individuals [79].

Follicular vitiligo is characterized by leukotrichia in the absence of depigmentation of the surrounding epidermis [80].

Segmental vitiligo presents with depigmented macules arranged in a segmental pattern that usually does not cross the midline. It is 10 times less common than other vitiligo types. The majority (87%) of the cases are detected before the age of 30 [76, 81]. Involvement of body hair (leukotrichia) and rapid onset are typical. Similar to NSV, the characteristic lesion is a nonscaly, chalky-white, amelanotic macule. In more than 50% of cases, the head is affected with the trigeminal dermatome most commonly involved [82]. The other common localizations are the trunk, limbs, extremities, and neck. In SV, the depigmentation progresses within the segment over a period of 6–24 months. After this period, the SV patch most often remains stable [76]. Segmental vitiligo is more refractory to treatment than other variants, possibly due to its more frequent association with leukotrichia and the deficiency of melanocyte reservoirs, which are involved in the repigmentation process [81].

Unclassifiable forms or undetermined vitiligo include focal vitiligo and mucosal vitiligo.

a. **Focal vitiligo:** Focal vitiligo is characterized by depigmented patches located in a small area without a typical segmental distribution and is classified as an undetermined type of vitiligo. A more definitive diagnosis can be made when the lesions have not evolved into non-segmental or segmental vitiligo after a period of 1–2 years [83].

b. **Mucosal vitiligo:** Involvement of one mucosal site is classified as indeterminate [84].

Vitiligo may show morphological variations, including trichrome, quadri-chrome vitiligo, penta-chrome vitiligo, blue vitiligo, and inflammatory vitiligo.

Trichrome vitiligo is characterized by the presence of an intermediate zone of hypopigmentation located between a vitiligo macule and normal pigmented surrounding skin. Hann et al. suggested that trichrome vitiligo a as a variant of unstable vitiligo [85].

Quadri-chrome vitiligo is characterized by the presence of perifollicular repigmentation in association with trichrome vitiligo [61].

Penta-chrome vitiligo is a rare vitiligo variant that shows blue-gray hyperpigmentation in addition to white, tan, and brown colors [61].

Blue vitiligo: Blue vitiligo is a unique variant of vitiligo presenting with asymptomatic bluish macules histopathologically corresponding to the presence of numerous dermal melanophages and the absence of epidermal melanocytes [86–88]

Inflammatory vitiligo: It is characterized by erythema on the areas of depigmentation and/or the border of the lesion [89]. These changes can be related to aggressive therapy.

3.2 Treatment

Various treatment strategies aiming to inhibit the immune response, reduce melanocyte destruction and reactivate residual melanocytes have been designed for the treatment of vitiligo. Choice of treatment is decided according to the subtype, the extent, distribution, and activity of the disease. The patient's age, phototype, effect on quality of life, and motivation for treatment should be considered in the treatment plan [7]. Treatments can be categorized as pharmacological, surgical, and physical treatments, which can be also used as a combination. Pharmacological treatments include topical and systemic steroids.

3.3 Pharmacological treatments

3.3.1 Topical treatments

3.3.1.1 Topical corticosteroids

Topical corticosteroids (TCS) are used as first-line treatments as monotherapy in localized vitiligo or in combination with phototherapy or other topical agents in generalized vitiligo. Topical corticosteroids (TCS) have anti-inflammatory and immunomodulating effects. Potent or ultrapotent corticosteroids may be used for the lesions on the body; midpotency topical corticosteroids should be used for the face, neck, intertriginous areas, and the lesions in children. Topical steroids can be used as daily or twice-daily applications in a cyclical fashion with treatment-free intervals (e.g., 1 week on then 1 week off for 6 months or application for 5 consecutive days followed by 2 days off) [90]. The treatment period should not be longer than 3 months because of adverse effects and tachyphylaxis. The advantages of topical steroid treatment therapy include wide availability, low cost, and efficacy. Recurrence after treatment cessation, and cutaneous side effects, such as skin atrophy, telangiectasia, and striae are the factors limiting corticosteroid use.

3.3.1.2 Topical calcineurin inhibitors

Calcineurin inhibitors can be effective in vitiligo treatment by regulating the altered cytokine network. This class of drugs includes tacrolimus and pimecrolimus. Calcineurin inhibitors bind to cytoplasmic protein macrophilin-12, forming a complex that blocks calcineurin. Calcineurin blockage inhibits the proliferation and activation of T cells, and the production of IL-2, IL-3, IL-4, IL-5, IFN-γ, and TNF-α, and suppresses the immune-mediated cutaneous inflammation [91]. Topical tacrolimus also stimulates melanocyte growth resulting in repigmentation [92]. Topical calcineurin inhibitors are generally the treatment of choice for face and neck vitiligo.

Tacrolimus 0.1% ointment was reported to be almost as efficacious as clobetasol propionate 0.05% ointment in a double-blind randomized controlled study [93–95]. Furthermore, a twice-weekly application of 0.1% tacrolimus ointment was shown to prevent the depigmentation of vitiligo patches that showed repigmentation after treatment [96]. Tacrolimus 0.1% ointment plus excimer laser was found to be more effective than placebo plus excimer laser [97].

Selective mode of action and absence of cutaneous atrophy and systemic absorption are some of the advantages of calcineurin inhibitors. No definite relationship between topical calcineurin inhibitor use and malignant tumors has been identified [93, 94, 98]. More studies about the possible risks of cutaneous and extracutaneous cancers are warranted.

3.3.1.3 Topical vitamin D derivatives

Vitamin D is synthesized in the epidermal keratinocytes under UVB light [99]. In addition to its role in regulating calcium and bone metabolism, vitamin D has immunoregulatory properties. The topical application of vitamin D has been shown to increase the number of L-3,4-dihydroxyphenylalanine-positive melanocytes [100]. Vitamin D analogs (calcipotriol and tacalcitol ointment) act in vitiligo by halting the local autoimmune process and activating melanocytic precursors and melanogenic pathways [101]. Lack of skin atrophy and easy application are the benefits of topical vitamin D derivatives. The use of calcipotriene may fasten the process of repigmentation and reduce overall cumulative exposure during phototherapy but appreciable repigmentation has not been obtained when used alone [81].

3.3.1.4 Pseudocatalase

Pseudocatalase is a complex, which is activated by ultraviolet B (UVB) radiation or natural sun and has been used to replace impaired catalase. Controversial results regarding the efficacy of pseudocatalase in vitiligo have been reported [102–105].

3.3.2 Systemic treatment

3.3.2.1 Systemic corticosteroids

Systemic corticosteroids can be administered as pulse therapy and short periods to stabilize the progression of vitiligo and induce repigmentation at the onset or early stages of the disease [106].

3.4 Physical treatment

3.4.1 Phototherapy

Phototherapy comprises narrowband UVB (NB UVB 311 nm), broadband UVB (BB UVB 290–320 nm), and photochemotherapy. UV plays a role in vitiligo treatment by regulating the activity of inflammatory cytokines, reducing the number of Langerhans cells, and polarizing the immune response toward Th2 profile. UV radiation also affects melanogenic cytokines involved in stimulating melanogenesis and the release of epidermal factors that stimulate melanocyte proliferation and migration [107]. Phototherapy shows better results if initiated early in the disease course [108]. It is used as first-line therapy in the treatment of extensive diseases. A combination of phototherapy with topical therapies, such as corticosteroids, tacrolimus, or calcipotriol, is also possible. Phototherapy cannot be used in patients with a history of xeroderma pigmentosum, systemic lupus erythematosus, porphyrias, skin viral infections, and previous treatment with photosensitizing agents. Since UV is a well-known cause of nonmelanoma skin cancers (NMSCs) and melanoma, concerns regarding whether repetitive UV light exposure during long-term phototherapy leads to an increase in the risk of photocarcinogenesis exist. However, in a meta-analysis, UV phototherapy has been reported to be a safe treatment for vitiligo with no significant risk of skin cancer [109].

3.4.2 Ultraviolet B narrowband

Narrowband UV (NB UVB) light (311 +/–2) is an effective and safe treatment modality in moderate or severe generalized vitiligo. In the last decade, NB UVB has become the first-line therapy for extensive progressive vitiligo due to its superiority to PUVA and relatively few side effects. It also has the advantage of being safely used in children during pregnancy or lactation.

Narrowband UV (NB UVB) light has been shown to have a greater response rate and treatment tolerance than PUVA and results in a better color match [110]. The repigmentation rate has been reported between 12.5% and 71.4% in various studies [111, 112]. Many therapeutic protocols are available, but the most commonly used NBUVB protocol is the application of the first dose of irradiation in doses between 0.075 J/cm^2 and 0.25 J/cm^2 and a dose increase by 20% in successive applications [113]. Treatment responsive patients can be treated with NBUVB for a maximum of 24 months. In children, the maximum allowable treatment duration is 12 months [114].

3.4.3 PUVA

Photochemotherapy (PUVA) is a treatment involving an exogenous photosensitizer mainly psoralen, followed by ultraviolet A (UVA) irradiation. UVA (320–400 nm). The mechanism of treatment is based on photoconjugation of psoralens in melanocyte DNA resulting in the proliferation of melanocytes, increased number of melanosomes, and their further transfer to keratinocytes. The psoralen derivative methoxsalen in an oral dose of 0.4 mg/kg body weight is administered 1–2 hours prior to irradiation. After treatment, UVA-blocking glasses and broad-spectrum sunscreens should be used [107]. PUVA is moderately effective in widespread vitiligo [115]. Complete repigmentation occurs in only 15–20% of patients treated with PUVA [115]. For patients with involvement of less than 20%, topical PUVA is indicated. For topical PUVA therapy methoxsalen, 0.1% is applied to vitiligo lesions 30–60 minutes before treatment.

3.4.4 Water bath PUVA

Water bath PUVA is a phototherapy method, in which the patient lies in a bathtub containing psoralen water for 15 min to provide the absorption of the drug on the skin before light therapy. This method is especially beneficial in children for whom oral medicines are not safe [116].

3.5 Laser therapy

The 308-nm excimer laser, formally named as the xenon chloride (XeCl) excimer (excited dimer) laser emits a monochromatic and coherent beam of narrow-band UVB (NbUVB) photons at 308 nm in short pulses focusing on the vitiliginous lesion [107]. These light sources are useful for safely treating small localized vitiligo lesions.

Fewer side effects compared to NBUVB occur since one lesion is treated at a time. Optimal esthetic results with minor contrast between normal and affected skin are obtained [107]. Long targeted treatment with an excimer laser promotes T-cell apoptosis and stimulates melanocyte development and progression along the hair follicle [117]. Two treatment sessions per week are administered for about 6 weeks. Treatment responses with an excimer laser are more rapid than NBUVB. Combination with topical tacrolimus or steroids results in enhanced treatment efficacy. Despite the lack of evidence, it is recommended that phototherapy should be continued for at least 3 months to halt the disease and induce repigmentation. The treatment can be continued for up to 1 year if there is a clinical response. Phototherapy should be stopped when there is no further response [117]. No data for cancer risk and long-term side effects are available, therefore, a cautious use of treatment is recommended.

4. Surgical treatment

Surgical therapies are reserved for patients with stable diseases who have failed to respond to medical treatments. Stable vitiligo is described as the absence of new lesions or an increase in the size of existing depigmented areas for at least 6 months. These treatment methods are typically used for the treatment refractory regions, such as the distal extremities (hands, feet, fingers, toes, palms, soles), elbows, knees, nipples, eyelids, and lips), [118, 119] and better results have been obtained in segmental vitiligo rather than generalized vitiligo [120, 121]. The Koebner phenomenon should be explained to all patients before performing surgical treatments. Several surgical options exist for the transplantation of melanocytes, including miniature punch grafting, suction blister grafting, transfer of noncultured epidermal suspensiosn, and transfer of cultured melanocytes [122]. Combination with UVB therapy results in more favorable treatment outcomes [4].

4.1 Cultured melanocytes

Cultured melanocytes can be transferred as pure-melanocyte suspensions or as melanocyte–keratinocyte co-cultures. Melanocyte–keratinocyte co-cultures have the advantage of containing melanogenic factors released by keratinocytes, which regulate melanocyte growth and differentiation. An autologous melanocyte culture is an effective tool in the treatment of vitiligo. Excellent repigmentation is achieved in 41% to 52% of patients and a good response in 7% to 19% [123, 124]. Several factors, including donor site selection and temperature of the donor tissue, are associated with an increase in the likelihood of successful melanocyte culturing [123]. Donor specimens can be harvested by biopsy or suction/cryo-induced blister method. Preparation of the recipient site can be performed by dermabrasion, suction/cryo-induced blister method Er:YAG laser or CO_2 laser. One of the most effective donor sites is the forearm because it has been found to produce melanocytes that proliferate fastest when cultured [122]. The major advantage of autologous melanocyte culture is its ability to treat a large vitiliginous area using tissue from only a small donor site [124].

4.2 Noncultured epidermal suspensions

In this technique, noncultured melanocyte/keratinocyte suspensions, which are prepared by 0.25% trypsin digestion of a thin piece of donor skin, are grafted to the recipient area. The procedure is performed by injecting the suspensions into blisters raised with liquid nitrogen or seeded onto dermabraded vitiligo lesions [107].

4.3 Minigrafting

Mini-punch grafting is the most commonly used technique for vitiligo repigmentation. With this technique, 2- to 4-mm punch grafts are harvested from a normally pigmented donor site of similar thickness [125, 126]. Generally, the grafts are harvested from the gluteus region or extensor surface of the thigh ("bikini area") [119]. Multiple punch biopsies that are the same size or 0.25 to 0.5 mm smaller than those taken from the donor site are taken from the recipient site [121]. The epidermis of the recipient site is often removed with phototherapy, dermabrasion, cryotherapy, or laser irradiation before the procedure [126]. The grafted area is covered with a petrolatum gauze dressing or a transparent adhesive tape and fixed with bandages for at least one week. Minigrafting method can also be used to treat difficult areas, such as lips. A cobblestoning appearance is a potential adverse effect of this method [125, 127]. The risk of cobblestoning appearance increases with the increasing size of the punch biopsies.

4.4 Suction blister grafting

Epidermal suction blister grafting is another useful tool available in the surgical management of vitiligo. In this technique, the formation of multiple epidermal blisters is promoted by a negative pressure apparatus which is applied to the normally pigmented donor site, producing 300 to 500 mmHg of pressure [128, 129]. Suction blisters can be simply produced by using the evacuated barrel of a syringe, which can generate negative pressure [130].

Pretreatment of the donor site with PUVA may increase the number of melanocytes available for transplantation [129]. The recipient site is prepared by removing the epidermis through induction of suction blisters, application of liquid nitrogen, PUVA, carbon dioxide laser, yttrium aluminum garnet laser, or dermabrasion. The roofs of the suction blisters formed at the donor site are subsequently removed and transferred to the newly prepared recipient site. The recipient site should be covered with a pressure bandage for 1 week, and the application of an antibiotic ointment at both sites is recommended.

4.5 Split thickness skin grafting

Grafts of the epidermis together with a part of the upper papillary dermis are implanted onto the recipient site. The grafts are harvested most commonly from the gluteal region or thigh. The procedure is performed by grafting of donor skin with a thickness of 0.1–0.2 mm using a hand dermatome or shaving blade fixed in a straight hemostat [129]. The grafts are implanted in recipient areas that have been prepared by dermabrasion or laser ablation. This technique is not suitable for vitiliginous lesions on the palms, soles, and skin folds.

4.6 Micropigmentation

Micropigmentation, also termed medical tattooing, can be a useful alternative treatment for treatment-resistant vitiligo. This technique is performed by the injection of pigment particles into the dermis, manually or with electrically driven needles [131, 132]. Tattooing is useful for sites with a poor rate of repigmentation, such as the lips, nipples, and distal fingers [131, 132].

4.7 Depigmentation

Depigmentation therapy is performed by the application of monobenzyl ether of hydroquinone (MBEH) to normally pigmented skin to induce selective melanocyte destruction. The exact mechanism of MBEH is not clearly known but it has been suggested that MBEH may act by the induction of necrotic changes in melanocyte plasma and nuclear membranes [133]. Typically, MBEH is applied twice daily for 6 to 18 months. A patch test should be performed to detect contact sensitivity to MBEH before treatment.

Depigmentation therapy is reserved for patients with the extensive or recalcitrant disease. Though there is no consensus regarding the stage of the disease that depigmentation should be initiated, it is usually offered for cases with involvement greater than 60% of body surface area or if visible areas, such as the face and hands, are affected [134].

The depigmentation therapy poses a permanent risk of acquiring sunburn. Patients should therefore be advised to minimize sun exposure and apply broad-spectrum sunscreens because of the possibility of the pigment relapse within a few weeks of treatment cessation on sun-exposed sites [135].

The possibility of carcinogenesis from hydroquinones is a debatable issue and the risk of carcinogenesis related to MBEH cannot be excluded [136].

4.8 Camouflage

The use of cosmetic camouflage on the face and other exposed areas can improve the quality of life for patients with vitiligo. Camouflage methods include cosmetic tattoos, dihydroxyacetone, general cosmetics, and various topical camouflage agents [137].

4.9 Novel treatments

4.9.1 Photodynamic therapy

The mechanism of photodynamic therapy (PDT) in vitiligo is based on the fundamental oxidative response. There are controversial results regarding the effect of PDT on vitiligo [138, 139]. Poor treatment responses may be related to the fact that melanin reflects this light length and PDT acts on oxidative stress, which is only one of the several mechanisms involved in the pathogenesis of vitiligo [139].

4.9.2 JAK inhibitors

JAK inhibitors have been offered as a novel treatment option for vitiligo. JAK inhibitors target the JAK/STAT pathway. JAK is involved in IFN-γ secretion. IFN-γ plays a key role in the pathogenesis of the disease and induces genes, including the T-cell chemokine receptor (CXCR3) and its multiple ligands, CXCL9, CXCL10, and CXCL11, which are upregulated in depigmented skin lesions. Activator of transcription (STAT)-1 signaling pathway leads to further recruitment of CXCR3+ CD8+ T cells, which causes melanocyte detachment and apoptosis [140].

JAK inhibitors, including ruxolitinib, baricitinib, and tofacitinib, have been found to be effective in vitiligo, and increasing treatment response is obtained with concomitant UV exposure. However, more studies regarding the ideal dosage of these drugs are required [140, 141]

4.9.3 Non-traditional treatments

Non-traditional treatments may be considered as an alternative for patients unresponsive to standard treatments. Vitamins, nutritional supplements, immunomodulators, khellin, topical and systemic phenylalanine, and herbal products are the most widely used [107]. Herbal formulations contain Psoralea corylifolia, black cumin, barberry root, and P leucotomos. Herbal products have anti-oxidative, anti-stress, immunoregulatory, and skin sensitizating effect to sunlight [116].

5. Conclusion

The etiopathogenesis of vitiligo has not been fully elucidated, despite the new discoveries in recent years. Integrated theory (Convergence theory) is currently the most accepted theory. No treatment option providing a definitive cure for vitiligo exists. Novel treatment modalities, such as JAK inhibitors and photodynamic therapy, enhanced the treatment perspective, while the results of these treatments need to be investigated by further studies.

Acknowledgements

I would like to thank Funda Kemeriz for her contribution to the preparation and design of the manuscript.

Conflict of interest statement

The author has no conflict of interest to declare.

Author details

Emine Müge Acar
VM Medicalpark Keçiören Hospital, Ankara, Turkey

*Address all correspondence to: drmugeacar@gmail.com

References

[1] Leung AKC, Lam JM, Leong KF, et al. Vitiligo: An updated narrative review. Current Pediatric Reviews. 2021;**17**(2):76-91

[2] Leone G, Pacifico A. Tacalcitol and narrow-band phototherapy in patients with vitiligo. Clinical Experimental Dermatology. 2006;**31**(2):200-205

[3] Wolff K, Goldsmith LA, Katz SI, Gilchrest BA, Paller AS, Leffell DJ. Fitzpatrick's Dermatology in General Medicine. 7th ed. Vol. Vol. I. USA: McGraw Hill; 2007. pp. 616-621

[4] Tonsi A. Vitiligo and its management update: A review. Pakistan Journal of Medical Science. 2004;**20**:242-247

[5] Mehta HR, Shah KC, Theodore C. Epidemiological study of vitiligo in Surat area, South Gujarat. The Indian Journal of Medical Research. 1973;**61**:145-154

[6] Halder RM, Nootheti PK. Ethnic skin disorders overview. Journal of the American Academy of Dermatology. 2003;**48**(6):143-148

[7] Bergqvist C, Ezzedine K. Vitiligo: A review. Dermatology. 2020;**236**(6):571-592

[8] Wang Y, Li S, Li C. Clinical features, immunopathogenesis, and therapeutic strategies in Vitiligo. Clinical Reviews in Allergy and Immunology. 2021;**61**(3):299-323

[9] Alikhan A, Felsten LM, Daly M, et al. Vitiligo: A comprehensive overview Part I. Introduction, epidemiology, quality of life, diagnosis, differential diagnosis, associations, histopathology, etiology, and work-up. Journal of the American Academy of Dermatology. 2011;**65**(3):473-491

[10] Ezzedine K, Eleftheriadou V, Whitton M, et al. Vitiligo. Lancet. 2015;**386**(9988):74-84

[11] Hamidizadeh N, Ranjbar S, Ghanizadeh A, et al. Evaluating prevalence of depression, anxiety and hopelessness in patients with vitiligo on an Iranian population. Health and Quality of Life Outcomes. 2020;**18**(1):1-7

[12] Stanescu AMA, Totan A, Mircescu D, et al. Assessment of suicidal behavior in dermatology (review). Experimental and Therapeutic Medicine. 2020;**20**(1):73-77

[13] Simons RE, Zevy DL, Jafferany M. Psychodermatology of vitiligo: Psychological impact and consequences. Dermatologic Therapy. 2020;**33**(3):e13418

[14] Mohammed GF, Gomaa AH, Al-Dhubaibi MS. Highlights in pathogenesis of vitiligo. World Journal of Clinical Cases. 2015;**3**:221

[15] Rezaei N, Gavalas NG, Weetman AP, et al. Autoimmunity as an aetiological factor in vitiligo. Journal of the European Academy of Dermatology and Venereology. 2007;**21**:865-876

[16] Buc M, Fazekasová H, Cechová E, et al. Occurrence rates of HLA-DRB1, HLA-DQB1, and HLA-DPB1 alleles in patients suffering fromvitiligo. European Journal of Dermatology. 1998;**8**:13-15

[17] Singh A, Sharma P, Kar HK, et al. HLA alleles and amino-acid signatures of the peptide-binding pockets of HLA molecules in vitiligo. The Journal of Investigative Dermatology. 2012;**132**:124-134

[18] Njoo MD, Westerhof W. Vitiligo: Pathogenesis and treatment. American

Journal of Clinical Dermatology. 2001;**2**:167-181

[19] Castanet J, Ortonne JP. Pathophysiology of vitiligo. Clinical Dermatology. 1997;**15**:845-851

[20] Alkhateeb A, Fain PR, Thody A, et al. Epidemiology of vitiligo and associated autoimmune diseases in Caucasian probands and their families. Pigment Cell Research. 2003;**16**:208-214

[21] Cunliffe W, Hall R, Newell J, et al. Vitiligo, thyroid disease and autoimmunity. The British Journal of Dermatology. 1968;**80**:135-139

[22] Amerio P, Tracanna M, De Remigis P, et al. Vitiligo associated with other autoimmune diseases: Polyglandular autoimmune syndrome types 3B+C and 4. Clinical and Experimental Dermatology. 2006;**31**:746-749

[23] Kemp EH, Emhemad S, Akhtar S, et al. Autoantibodies against tyrosine hydroxylase in patients with non-segmental (generalised) vitiligo. Experimental Dermatology. 2011;**20**:35-40

[24] Kemp EH, Gawkrodger DJ, Watson PF, et al. Immunoprecipitation of melanogenic enzyme autoantigens with vitiligo sera: Evidence for cross-reactive autoantibodies to tyrosinase and tyrosinase-related protein-2 (TRP-2). Clinical and Experimental Immunology. 1997;**109**:495-500

[25] Kemp EH, Waterman EA, Gawkrodger DJ, et al. Autoantibodies to tyrosinase-related protein-1 detected in the sera of vitiligo patients using a quantitative radiobinding assay. The British Journal of Dermatology. 1998;**139**:798-805

[26] Baharav E, Merimski O, Shoenfeld Y, et al. Tyrosinase as an autoantigen in patients with vitiligo. Clinical and Experimental Immunology. 1996;**105**:84

[27] Passeron T, Ortonne JP. Physiopathology and genetics of vitiligo. Journal of Autoimmune. 2005;**25**:63-68

[28] Oyarbide-Valencia K, van den Boorn JG, et al. Therapeutic implications of autoimmune vitiligo T cells. Autoimmunity Reviews. 2006;**5**:486-492

[29] Zhou L, Li K, Shi YL, Hamzavi I, et al. Systemic analyses of immunophenotypes of peripheral T cells in non-segmental vitiligo: Implication of defective natural killer T cells. Pigment Cell & Melanoma Research. 2012;**25**:602-611

[30] Palermo B, Campanelli R, Garbelli S, et al. Specific cytotoxic T lymphocyte responses againstMelan-A/MART1, tyrosinase and gp100 in vitiligo by the use of major histocompatibility complex/peptide tetramers: The role of cellular immunity in the etiopathogenesis of vitiligo. The Journal of Investigative Dermatology. 2001;**117**(2):326-332

[31] Ogg GS, Dunbar PR, Romero P, et al. High frequency of skin-homing melanocyte-specific cytotoxic T lymphocytes in autoimmune vitiligo. The Journal of Experimental Medicine. 1998;**21**:1203-1208

[32] Taher ZA, Lauzon G, Maguiness S, et al. Analysis of interleukin-10 levels in lesions of vitiligo following treatment with topical tacrolimus. The British Journal of Dermatology. 2009;**161**:654-659

[33] Speeckaert R, Speeckaert MM, van Geel N. Why treatments do(n't) work in vitiligo: An autoinflammatory

perspective. Autoimmunity Reviews. 2015;**14**:332-340

[34] Gauthier Y, Cario-Andre M, Lepreux S, et al. Melanocyte detachment non lesional skin of patients with generalized vitiligo. The British Journal of Dermatology. 2003;**148**:95-101

[35] Gauthier Y, Cario Andre M, Taieb A. A critical appraisal of vitiligo etiologic theories. Is melanocyte loss a melanocytorrhagy? Pigment Cell Research. 2003;**16**:322-332

[36] Le Poole IC, van den Wijngaard RM. Tenascin is overexpressed in vitiligo lesional skin and inhibits melanocyte adhesion. British Journal of Dermatology. 1997;**137**:171-178

[37] Dell'Anna ML, Maresca V, Briganti S, et al. Mitochondrial impairment in peripheral blood mononuclear cells during the active phase of vitiligo. The Journal of Investigative Dermatology. 2001;**117**(4):908-913

[38] Maresca V, Roccella M, Roccella F, et al. Increased sensitivity to peroxidative agents as a possible pathogenic factor of melanocyte damage in vitiligo. The Journal of Investigative Dermatology. 1997;**109**(3):310-313

[39] Jimbow K, Chen H, Park JS, et al. Increased sensitivity of melanocytes to oxidative stress and abnormal expression of tyrosinase related protein in vitiligo. The British Journal of Dermatology. 2001;**144**(1):55-65

[40] Speeckaert R, Dugardin J, Lambert J, et al. Critical appraisal of the oxidative stress pathway in vitiligo: A systematic review and meta-analysis. Journal of the European Academy of Dermatology and Venereology. 2018;**32**(7):1089-1098

[41] Sahera S, Reddy YV, Kumar DS. A rare case report of Vitiligo Vulgaris in pediatric patient in tertiary care hospital. IOSR Journal of Dental Medicine Science. 2020;**20**:42-47

[42] Richmond JM, Frisoli ML, Harris JE. Innate immune mechanisms in vitiligo: Danger from within. Current Opinion in Immunology. 2013;**25**(6):676-682

[43] Dell'Anna ML, Ottaviani M, Albanesi V, et al. Membrane lipid alterations as a possible basis for melanocyte degeneration in vitiligo. The Journal of Investigative Dermatology. 2007;**127**(5):1226-1233

[44] Dell'Anna ML, Urbanelli S, Mastrofrancesco A, et al. Alterations of mitochondria in peripheral blood mononuclear cells of vitiligo patients. Pigment Cell Research. 2003:553-559

[45] Prota G. The role of peroxidase in melanogenesis revisited. Pigment Cell Research. 1992;**2**:25-31

[46] Schallreuter KU, Elwary SM, Gibbons NC, et al. Activation/deactivation of acetylcholinesterase by H2O2: More evidence for oxidative stress in vitiligo. Biochemical and Biophysical Research Communications. 2004;**315**(2):502-508

[47] Schallreuter KU, Wood JM, Berger J. Low catalase levels in the epidermis of patients with vitiligo. The Journal of Investigative Dermatology. 1991;**97**(6):1081-1085

[48] Lerner AB. Vitiligo. The Journal of Investigative Dermatology. 1959;**32**:285-310

[49] Wu CS, Yu HS, Chang HR, et al. Cutaneous blood flow and adrenoceptor response increase in segmental-type

vitiligo lesions. Journal of Dermatological Science. 2000;**23**:53-62

[50] Rateb AAH, Azzam OA, Rashed LA, et al. The role of nerve growth factor in the pathogenesis of vitligo. Journal of the Egyptian Womens Dermatologic Society. 2005;**1**:18-24

[51] Morrone A, Picardo M, Luca CD, et al. Catecholamines and vitiligo. Pigment Cell Research. 1992;**5**:65-69

[52] Stokes PE, Sikes CR. The hypothalamic-pituitary-adrenocortical axis in major depression. Neurologic Clinics. 1988;**6**:1-19

[53] Akbayir N, Gökdemir G, Mansur T, et al. Is there any relationship between hepatitis C virus and vitiligo?J. Clinics in Gastroenterology. 2004;**38**(9):815-817

[54] Akcan Y, Kavak A, Sertbas Y, et al. The low seropositivity of hepatitis B virus in vitiligo patients. Journal of the European Academy of Dermatology and Venereology. 2006;**20**:110-111

[55] Toker SC, Sarycaoglu H, Karadogan SK, Mistik R, Baskan EB, Tunaly S. Is there any relation between vitiligo and cytomegalovirus? Journal of the European Academy of Dermatology and Venereology. 2007;**21**:141-142

[56] İverson MV. Hypothesis. Vitiligo virus. Pigment Cell Research. 2000;**13**:281-282

[57] Duvic M, Rapini R, Hoots WK, et al. Human immunodeficiency virus-associated vitiligo: Expression of autoimmunity with immunodeficiency? Journal of the American Academy of Dermatology. 1987;**17**:656-662

[58] Erf GF, Bersi TK, Wang X, et al. Herpesvirus connection in the expression of autoimmune vitiligo in Smyth line chickens. Pigment Cell Research. 2001;**14**:40-46

[59] Niamba P, Traoré A, Taïeb A. Vitiligo in a black patient associated with HIV infection and repigmentation under antiretroviral therapy. Annals of Dermatology and Venereology. 2007;**134**:272-273

[60] Bagherani N, Yaghoobi R, Omidian M. Hypothesis: Zinc can be effective in treatment of vitiligo. Indian Journal of Dermatology. 2011;**56**:480-484

[61] Yaghoobi R, Omidian M, Bagherani N. Vitiligo: A review of the published work. The Journal of Dermatology. 2011;**38**:419-431

[62] Liu T, Luo X, Li ZH, et al. Zinc-α2-glycoprotein 1 attenuates non-alcoholic fatty liver disease by negatively regulating tumour necrosis factor-α. World Journal of Gastroenterology. 2019;**25**(36):5451-5468

[63] El-Rifaie A, Gohary YM, Abd-El Aziz GM, et al. Zinc-alpha2-Glycoprotein (ZAG): A new deficiency in Vitiligo patients. Skinmed. 2019;**17**:248-253

[64] Gordon PR, Mansur CP, Gilchrest BA. Regulation of human melanocyte growth, dendricity, and melanization by keratinocyte derived factors. The Journal of Investigative Dermatology. 1989;**92**:565-572

[65] Hassan MI, Waheed A, Yadav S, et al. Zinc alpha 2-glycoprotein: A multidisciplinary protein. Molecular Cancer Research. 2008;**6**:892-906

[66] Azzam OA, El Sherbeiny MH, Shaker OG, et al. Assessment of serum zinc, serum, and tissue zinc α2-glycoprotein levels in vitiligo: A pilot study. JEWDS. 2020;**17**(2):91

[67] Boissy RE, Liu YY, Medrano EE, et al. Structural aberration of the rough endoplasmic reticulum and melanosome compartmentalization in long-term cultures of melanocytes from vitiligo patients. The Journal of Investigative Dermatology. 1991;**97**:395-404

[68] Norris A, Todd C, Graham A, et al. The expression of the c-kit receptor by epidermal melanocytes may be reduced in vitiligo. The British Journal of Dermatology. 1996;**134**:299-306

[69] van den Wijngaard R, Wankowicz-Kalinska A, Le Poole C, et al. Local immune response in skin of generalized vitiligo patients. Destruction of melanocytes is associated with the prominent presence of CLA+ T cells at the perilesional site. Laboratory Investigation. 2000;**80**:1299-1309

[70] Boissy RE. Histology of vitiliginous skin. In: Hann S, Nordlund JJ, editors. Vitiligo. 1st ed. Oxford: Blackwell Science Ltd; 2008. pp. 23-34

[71] Tschopp J, Martinon F, Burns K. NALPs: A novel protein family involved in inflammation. Nature Reviews. Molecular Cell Biology. 2003;**4**:95-104

[72] Lee AY, Youm YH, Kim NH, et al. Keratinocytes in the depigmented epidermis of vitiligo are more vulnerable to trauma (suction) than keratinocytes in the normally pigmented epidermis, resulting in their apoptosis. The British Journal of Dermatology. 2004;**151**:995-1003

[73] Bondanza S, Maurelli R. Keratinocyte cultures from involved skin in vitiligo patients show an impaired in vitro behaviour. Pigment Cell Research. 2007;**20**(4):288-300

[74] Le Poole IC, Das PK, Van Den Wijngaard RM, et al. Review of the etiopathomechanism of vitiligo: A convergence theory. Experimental Dermatology. 1993;**2**(4):145-153

[75] Osman AM, Elkordufani Y, Abdullah MA, et al. The psychological impact of vitiligo in adult Sudanese patients. African Journal of Psychiatry. 1993;**12**(4)

[76] Hann SK, Lee HJ. Segmental vitiligo: Clinical findings in 208 patients. Journal of the American Academy of Dermatology. 1996;**35**(5):671-674

[77] Ezzedine K, Diallo A, Léauté-Labrèze C, et al. Halo naevi and leukotrichia are strong predictors of the passage to mixed vitiligo in a subgroup of segmental vitiligo. The British Journal of Dermatology. 2012;**166**(3):539-544

[78] Falabella R, Escobar CE, Carrascal E, et al. Leukoderma punctata. Journal of the American Academy of Dermatology. 1988;**18**(3):485-494

[79] Ezzedine K, Mahe A, van Geel N, et al. Hypochromic vitiligo: Delineation of a new entity. The British Journal of Dermatology. 2015;**172**(3):716-721

[80] Gan EY, Cario-Andre M, Pain C, et al. Follicular vitiligo: A report of 8 cases. Journal of the American Academy of Dermatology. 2016;**74**(6):1178-1184

[81] Rodrigues M, Ezzedine K, Hamzavi I, et al. Vitiligo Working Group. Current and emerging treatments for vitiligo. Journal of the American Academy of Dermatology. 2017;**77**(1):17-29

[82] Silverberg NB, Charona MI, Arrunátegui A, Falabella R, Alzate A. An epidemiologic case-control study in a population with vitiligo. Journal of the American Academy of Dermatology. 1995;**33**(4):621-625

[83] Lommerts JE, Schilder Y, de Rie MA. Focal vitiligo: Long-term follow-up of 52 cases. Journal of European Academic Dermatology. 2016;**30**(9):1550-1554

[84] Ezzedine K, Lim HW, Suzuki T, et al. Vitiligo Global Issue Consensus Conference Panelists. Revised classification/nomenclature of vitiligo and related issues: The Vitiligo Global Issues Consensus Conference. Pigment Cell & Melanoma Research. 2012;**25**(3):E1-E13

[85] Hann SK, Kim YS, Yoo JH, et al. Clinical and histopathologic characteristics of trichrome vitiligo. Journal of the American Academy of Dermatology. 2000;**42**(4):589-596

[86] Zhang JA, Yu JB, Lv Y, et al. Blue vitiligo following intralesional injection of psoralen combined with ultraviolet B radiation therapy. Clinical and Experimental Dermatology. 2015;**40**:301-304

[87] Ivker R, Goldaber M, Buchness MR. Blue vitiligo. Journal of the American Academy of Dermatology. 1994;**30**:829-831

[88] Ankad B, Nikam B, Jaju P. Blue vitiligo: A dermoscopic perspective. Indian Journal of Dermatology, Venereology and Leprology. 2019;**85**(6):634-637

[89] Soro LA, Gust AJ, Purcell SM. Inflammatory vitiligo versus hypopigmented mycosis fungoides in a 58-year-old Indian female. Indian Dermatology Online Journal. 2013;**4**(4):321

[90] Stinco G, Trevisan G, Buligan C, et al. Narrow band-ultraviolet B versus clobetasol propionate foam in the treatment of vitiligo: A retrospective study. Dermatologic Therapy. 2013;**3**:95-105

[91] Gutfreund K, Bienias W, Szewczyk A, et al. Topical calcineurin inhibitors in dermatology. Part I: Properties, method and effectiveness of drug use. Postepy Dermatology Alergology. 2013;**3**:165-169

[92] Lan CC, Chen GS, Chiou MH, et al. FK506 promotes melanocyte and melanoblast growth and creates a favourable milieu for cell migration via keratinocytes: Possible mechanisms of how tacrolimus ointment induces repigmentation in patients with vitiligo. The British Journal of Dermatology. 2005;**153**(3):498-505

[93] Schneeweiss S, Doherty M, Zhu S, et al. Topical treatments with pimecrolimus, tacrolimus and medium- to high- potency corticosteroids, and risk of lymphoma. Dermatology. 2009;**219**:7-21

[94] Luger T, Boguniewicz M, Carr W, et al. Pimecrolimus in atopic dermatitis: Consensus on safety and the need to allow use in infants. Pediatric Allergy and Immunology. 2015;**26**(4):306-315

[95] Lepe V, Moncada B, Castanedo-Cazares JP, et al. A double-blind randomized trial of 0.1% tacrolimus vs 0.05% clobetasol for the treatment of childhood vitiligo. Achieves in Dermatology. 2003;**139**:867-897

[96] Cavalié M, Ezzedine K, Fontas E, et al. Maintenance therapy of adult vitiligo with 0.1% tacrolimus ointment: A randomized, double blind, placebo-controlled study. The Journal of Investigative Dermatology. 2015;**135**:970-974

[97] Kawalek AZ, Spencer JM, Phelps RG. Combined excimer laser and topical

tacrolimus for the treatment of vitiligo: A pilot study. Dermatologic Surgery. 2004;**30**:130-135

[98] Arellano FM, Wentworth CE, Arana A, et al. Risk of lymphoma following exposure to calcineurin inhibitors and topical steroids in patients with atopic dermatitis. The Journal of Investigative Dermatology. 2007;**127**:808-816

[99] Lehmann B, Querings K. Reichrath J "Vitamin D and skin: New aspects for dermatology.". Experimental Dermatology. 2004;**13**:11-15

[100] AlGhamdi K, Kumar A, Moussa N. The role of vitamin D in melanogenesis with an emphasis on vitiligo. Indian Journal of Dermatology, Venereology and Leprology. 2013:79(6)

[101] Oh SH, Kim M. Vitamin D and Vitiligo. London: INTECH Open Access Publisher; 2011

[102] Gawkrodger DJ. Pseudocatalase and narrowband ultraviolet B for vitiligo: Clearing the picture. The British Journal of Dermatology. 2009;**161**:721-728

[103] Yuksel EP, Aydin F, Senturk N, et al. Comparison of the efficacy of narrow band ultraviolet B and narrow band ultraviolet B plus topical catalase-superoxide dismutase treatment in vitiligo patients. European Journal of Dermatology. 2009;**19**:341-344

[104] Bakis-Petsoglou S, Le Guay JL, et al. randomized, double-blinded, placebo-controlled trial of pseudocatalase cream and narrowband ultraviolet B in the treatment of vitiligo. The British Journal of Dermatology. 2009;**161**:910-917

[105] Sanclemente G, Garcia JJ, Zuleta JJ, et al. A double-blind, randomized trial of 0.05% betamethasone vs. topical catalase/dismutase superoxide in vitiligo. Journal of the European Academy of Dermatology and Venereology. 2008;**22**:1359-1364

[106] Kim SM, Lee HS, Hann SK. The efficacy of low-dose oral corticosteroids in the treatment of vitiligo patients. International Journal of Dermatology. 1999;**38**:546-550

[107] Birlea SA, Spritz RA, Norris DA. Vitiligo. In: Goldsmith LA, Katz SI, Gilchrest BA, Paller AS, Lefell DJ, Wolff K, editors. Fitzpatrick's Dermatology in General Medicine. 8th ed. McGraw Hill; 2012. pp. 792-803

[108] Bansal S, Sahoo B, Garg V. Psoralen–narrowband UVB phototherapy for the treatment of vitiligo comparison to narrowband UVB alone. Photodermatology, Photoimmunology & Photomedicine. 2013;**29**(6):311-317

[109] Wu YH, Chou CL, Chang HC. Risk of skin cancer after ultraviolet phototherapy in patients with vitiligo: A systematic review and meta-analysis. Clinical and Experimental Dermatology. 2022;**47**(4):692-699

[110] Falabella R, Barona MI. Update on skin repigmentation therapies in vitiligo. Pigment Cell & Melanoma Research. 2009;**22**(1):42-65

[111] Kanwar AJ, Dogra S, Parsad D, et al. Narrow-band UVB for the treatment of vitiligo: An emerging effective and well-tolerated therapy. International Journal of Dermatology. 2005;**44**(1):57-60

[112] Chen GY, Hsu MML, Tai HK, et al. Narrow-band UVB treatment of vitiligo in Chinese. The Journal of Dermatology. 2005;**32**(10):793-800

[113] Hercogová J, Buggiani G, Prignano F, et al. A rational approach

to the treatment of vitiligo and other hypomelanoses. In: Lotti T, Thiers BH, editors. Pigmentary Disorders. Vol. 25. 2007. pp. 383-392

[114] Njoo MD, Westerhof W, Bos JD, et al. The development of guidelines for the treatment of vitiligo. Archives of Dermatology. 1999;**135**:1514-1521

[115] Kwok YKC, Anstey AV, Hawk JLM. Psoralen photochemotherapy (PUVA) is only moderately effective in widespread vitiligo: A 10-year retrospective study. Clinical and Experimental Dermatology. 2002;**27**(2):104-110

[116] Tahir MA, Pramod K, Ansari SH, et al. Current remedies for vitiligo. Autoimmunity Reviews. 2010;**9**(7):516-520

[117] Daniel BS, Wittal R. Vitiligo treatment update. Australian Journal of Dermatology. 2015;**56**(2):85-92

[118] Kumar P. Autologous punch grafting for vitiligo of the palm. Dermatologic Surgery. 2005;**31**:368-370

[119] Mulekar SV, Al Issa A, Al EA. Treatment of vitiligo on difficult-to-treat sites using autologous noncultured cellular grafting. Dermatologic Surgery. 2009;**35**:66-71

[120] Mulekar SV. Melanocyte–keratinocyte cell transplantation for stable vitiligo. International Journal of Dermatology. 2003;**42**(2):132-136

[121] Gupta S, Kumar B. Epidermal grafting in vitiligo: Influence of age, site of leşion, and type of disease on outcome. Journal of the American Academy of Dermatology. 2003;**49**(1):99-104

[122] Patel NS, Paghdal KV. Cohen GF Advanced treatment modalities for vitiligo. Dermatologic Surgery. 2012;**38**(3):381-391

[123] Czajkowski R, Placek W, Drewa T, et al. Autologous cultured melanocytes in vitiligo treatment. Dermatologic Surgery. 2012;**33**(9):1027-1036

[124] Pianigiani E, Risulo M, Andreassi A, Taddeucci P, et al. Autologous epidermal cultures and narrow-band ultraviolet B in the surgical treatment of vitiligo. Dermatologic Surgery. 2005;**31**:155

[125] Lahiri K, Malakar S, Sarma N, et al. Repigmentation of vitiligo with punch grafting and narrow-band UV-B (311 nm)— a prospective study. International Journal of Dermatology. 2006;**45**:649-655

[126] Sachdev M, Shankar DS. Dermatologic surgery: Pulsed erbium: YAG laser-assisted autologous epidermal punch grafting in vitiligo. International Journal of Dermatology. 2000;**39**:868-871

[127] Gupta S, Jain VK, Saraswat PK, et al. Suction blister epidermal grafting versus punch skin grafting in recalcitrant and stable vitiligo. Dermatologic Surgery. 1999;**25**:955-958

[128] Njoo MD, Westerhof W, Bos JD, et al. A systematic review of autologous transplantation methods in vitiligo. Archives of Dermatology. 1998;**134**:1543-1549

[129] Rusfianti M, Wirohadidjodjo YW. Dermatosurgical techniques for repigmentation of vitiligo. International Journal of Dermatology. 2006;**45**:411-417

[130] Hasegawa T, Suga Y, Ikejima A, et al. Suction blister grafting with CO(2) laser resurfacing of the graft recipient site for vitiligo. The Journal of Dermatology. 2007;**34**:490-492

[131] Garg G, Thami GP. Micropigmentation: Tattooing for medical purposes. Dermatologic Surgery. 2005;**31**:928-931

[132] Mutalik S, Ginzburg A. Surgical management of stable vitiligo: A review with personal experience. Dermatologic Surgery. 2000;**26**(3):248-254

[133] Hariharan V, Klarquist J, Reust MJ, et al. Monobenzyl ether of hydroquinone and 4-tertiary butyl phenol activate markedly different physiological responses in melanocytes: Relevance to skin depigmentation. The Journal of Investigative Dermatology. 2010;**1**:211-220

[134] Alghamdi KM, Kumar A. Depigmentation therapies for normal skin in vitiligo universalis. Journal of the European Academy of Dermatology and Venereology. 2011;**25**:749-757

[135] Njoo MD, Vodegel RM, Westerhof W. Depigmentation therapy in vitiligo universalis with topical 4-methoxyphenol and the Q-switched ruby laser. Journal of the American Academy of Dermatology. 2000;**42**:760-769

[136] Gawkrodger DJ, Ormerod AD, Shaw L, et al. Guideline for the diagnosis and management of vitiligo. The British Journal of Dermatology. 2008;**159**(5):1051-1076

[137] Hossain C, Porto DA, Hamzavi I. Camouflaging agents for Vitiligo patients. Journal of Drugs in Dermatology. 2016;**15**(4):38

[138] Zhang Y, Lin H, Guo X, et al. A case series pilot study on the combination of 5-aminolevulinic acid and photodynamic therapy (ALA-PDT) for treatment of vitiligo. Anais Brasileiros de Dermatologia. 2018;**93**:539-545

[139] Rahimi H, Zeinali R, Tehranchinia Z. Photodynamic therapy of vitiligo: A pilot study. Photodiagnosis and Photodynamic Therapy. 2021;**36**:102439

[140] Qi F, Liu F, Gao L. Janus kinase inhibitors in the treatment of vitiligo: A review. Frontiers in Immunology. 2021;**12**:790125

[141] Relke N, Gooderham M. The use of Janus kinase inhibitors in vitiligo: A review of the literature. Journal of Cutaneous Medicine and Surgery. 2019;**23**(3):298-306

Chapter 4

Psychological Impact of Vitiligo

Nayra Merino, Mónica Fumero, Maria Eugenia Gaviño and Marta García-Bustinduy

Abstract

Vitiligo is a depigmentation disorder with a high psychological impact. It affects 0.5–2% of the population worldwide. Psychological comorbidities associated with vitiligo are feelings of stigmatization, adjustment disorders, sleep disturbance, relationship difficulties, including sexual dysfunction and avoidance or restriction behavior. Depression, anxiety, and alexithymia have been associated too and we have several studies in this way, they will be included in the chapter. Female sex, visible or genital lesions, age < 30 years, and greater body surface area involvement are risk factors to develop psychological comorbidities. Psychological test (HADS, TAS-20, DLQI, or BDI-II) could be useful to assess these patients and to decide the better therapeutical approach.

Keywords: Vitiligo, psychological, anxiety, depression, alexithymia, stigmatization, quality of life

1. Introduction

Depression and anxiety are reported as the most frequent psychosocial comorbidities in vitiligo patients. The following psychological comorbidities have been reported in more than 50% of these subjects in any study: depression, major depression disorder, anxiety, social phobia, feelings of stigmatization, adjustment disorders, sleep disturbances, avoidance and restriction behavior, self-consciousness, emotional impaired, relationship difficulties, and cognitive impairment. Psychosocial comorbidities reported in more than 25% of patients include coexisting depression and anxiety, sexual dysfunction, alexithymia, anger, suicidal thoughts, and dysthymic disorders [1]. Therefore, it is important to know the aspects that could aggravate the course of the disease, so we are going to list all of them.

1.1 Race/ethnicity

People with darker skin present more stigmatization and greater discrimination, since the contrast between normal and depigmented skin is much more evident. For this reason, psychosocial issues in this type of patient are very common [2].

1.2 Extension and localization of vitiligo lesions

Vitiligo lesions can appear in any part of the body, taking more or less extension.

As expected, when vitiligo affects a greater part of the body, the impact on the patient's life quality is much more severe.

Is important to highlight that vitiligo does not affect equally when lesions are more visible since the more visible the lesions are to society, the more repercussions it has in the life quality of the individuals. In this case, the areas with greater exposure and psychological affectation usually are the face (**Figure 1**) and hands (**Figure 2**), without forgetting sensitive areas, such as genitals. With regard to this last part, when vitiligo is present in genitals, most of the time it is not reported to specialists because of embarrassment or stigmatization that it could be related to a sexually transmitted disease [3].

We know that vitiligo is usually asymptomatic, so the negative impact in the life quality is related to several psychological issues, such as a decrease in self-confidence or failure in social relationships [4].

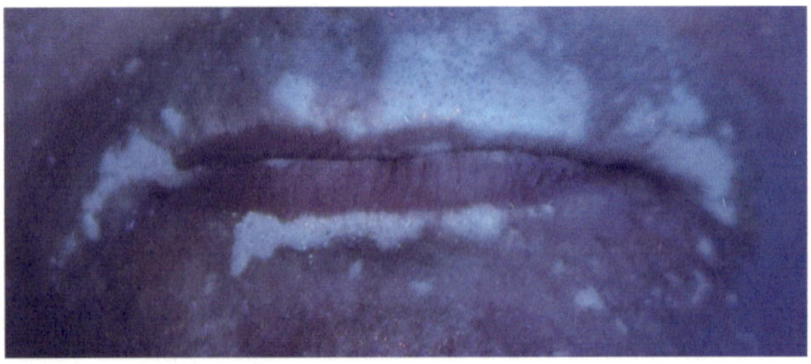

Figure 1.
Vitiligo lesions on the face (perioral distribution) with wood light.

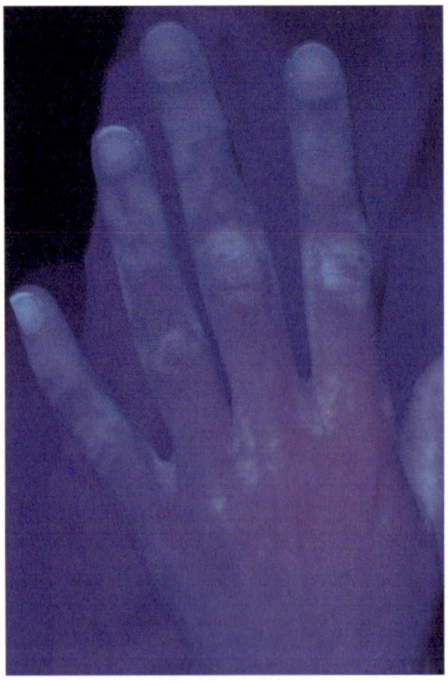

Figure 2.
Vitiligo lesions on the dorsum of the left hand with wood light.

1.3 Gender

There are skin diseases that do not affect equally between sexes. The social stigma to which they are bound and the lack of information from society in general lead us to "a weaker sex."

Like in other skin disorders, such as alopecia, women who suffer from vitiligo have higher stress level than men. In addition to this, women manifest more hopelessness feelings [5].

1.4 Physical appearance

Nowadays, many cultures and societies give great importance to appearance, esthetic, and pigmentation. Therefore, any condition that affects appearance can lead to loss of privileges and opportunities.

The visibility of vitiligo, like other skin disorders, can affect considerably in terms of self-confidence. Patients who suffer from any skin disease like acne or vitiligo have experienced the feeling of being ugly or unattractive [6].

2. Psychological impairment and vitiligo

2.1 Stigmatization and quality of life

Vitiligo is more than a biological disorder. Several psychological and social disturbances have been described in these patients, which could interfere with their interpersonal relationships. The location and visibility of the lesions, as well as their size, are reported as a cause of suffering, not only for esthetic reasons but because of the discriminatory and stigmatizing views received in different social areas [1]. Stigmatization and discrimination are "justified" as a sign of fear of getting the disease. A negative image of themselves is usually associated with these patients. Thus, several resources to hide or camouflage the signs of vitiligo have been used by them, such as the use of makeup or the adaptation of their clothing. In addition, these subjects develop avoidance behaviors. All of this can lead to social isolation and low self-esteem [7].

Many civilizations and global societies assign great importance to physical appearance, esthetics, and skin pigmentation. Any condition that involves the esthetic appearance may lead to a loss of privileges and opportunities, and could disturb the professional career as well as personal and social interactions. This effect on self-esteem and the perception of beauty transcends race, age, gender, and socioeconomic status [3].

The impact of vitiligo on patients' quality of life has been estimated in global populations with variable results. However, most of the results corroborate the negative impact of the disease on the self-esteem and quality of life of these patients [3]. When the affected body surface is greater than 25%, studies suggest a significant deterioration in the quality of life [8]. On the other hand, multiple studies have reported that lesions that affect more visible areas, such as the face or hands, and more sensitive areas, such as the genitals, have a more severe impact on the quality of life of these patients. Patients with involvement in the genital areas often do not consult doctors due to embarrassment or even the stigmatization that it could be related to a sexually transmitted disease. In addition, these patients may present sexual dysfunction, with equal frequency in male and female patients. Therefore, genital involvement and generalized vitiligo are significant risk factors that affect the sexual life of patients [3].

By gender, studies have reported more difficulties to accept the disease in women, secondary to its esthetic dysfunction, showing more troubles in social adaptation. A relationship between culture and the psychological burden of vitiligo has been reported. In addition, in young single women who live in a country with arranged marriages, vitiligo decreases the chances of marriage and in married women who develop the disease, the chance of divorce is increased. On the other hand, it is often assumed that the psychological disturbance is greater in racial or ethnic groups with darker skin [1, 3, 9].

The 25–38% of vitiligo patients are children. As in adults, several studies suggest that children experience a substantial disturbance related to vitiligo with a worse quality of life. Children and parents consider the face and legs as the most stigmatized areas. A large extension (BSA >25%) was associated with self-consciousness, fear, and bullying [8]. Negative childhood experiences may develop more problems in social relationships in adult life [10]. Furthermore, the quality of life of relatives has also been evaluated, and the findings suggest that parents of children with vitiligo experience significant psychological trauma and altered quality of life [3].

2.2 Alexithymia and vitiligo

Alexithymia is not only related to psychosomatic illnesses. Nowadays, it is considered as a risk factor for many medical and psychiatric illnesses [11]. Historically, much of the attention regarding alexithymia has focused on its overlap with autism spectrum disorder (ASD). The prevalence of alexithymia in ASD has been reported to be up to 63%, compared with the general population [12]. It is defined as a difficulty in differentiating, describing, distinguishing, or expressing one's own feelings and those of others. Therefore, alexithymic subjects have a lower capacity to cope with stress. Psychological stress is known to be an important trigger in the onset or exacerbation of many dermatological diseases, including vitiligo [11].

Alexithymia is defined by three main features:

- Difficulty in identifying feelings, and, further, difficulty distinguishing between feelings and the bodily sensations of emotional arousal.

- Difficulty in describing feelings to other people.

- Restricted imaginative processes and externally oriented cognitive style.

The highly sensitive to physical stimuli is the link between alexithymia, a psychological construct, and physical illness. This high sensitivity may increase their likelihood of experiencing somatic symptoms during long periods of time. Alexithymia is often accompanied by mind-body mismatch and poor quality of social relationships, which may result in psychological distress and negative emotions. Such negative emotions and the physical sensations that accompany them (e.g., increased heart rate, sweating) tend to be confused with symptoms of illness. If this situation is prolonged in time, an intensified nervous system response from the neuroendocrine system could be arisen, further contributing to somatic disease [12].

Beyond somatic illness, alexithymia is related to other mental diseases. In fact, up to 58%, 51%, and 49% of alexithymic patients appear to suffer anxiety, depression, and addictive behaviors, respectively. Even more, higher levels of alexithymia appear to be associated with more severe manifestations of psychiatric illness [12].

An important interaction between alexithymia and skin disease has been reported. A 2008 systematic review concluded that alexithymia, which is related to changes in sympathetic activity, immunity, and brain activity, is associated with a number of dermatological diseases. In the findings reported up to September 2008, it was concluded that patients with alopecia areata, vitiligo, and urticaria have a higher prevalence and severity of alexithymia compared with healthy controls. For patients with psoriasis and atopic dermatitis, the results were contradictory, so that some studies suggested a higher prevalence of alexithymia in patients with these diagnoses and others did not [13].

More recently, in another systematic review published in 2022, the evidence accumulated after September 1, 2008, up to March 12, 2021, is reviewed, to better understand the relationship between alexithymia and dermatological diseases. Due to the inability of these people to understand, describe and specify emotions, which can create a significant barrier to self-control (essential in dermatology given the chronicity of many conditions), the impact of alexithymia on the burden of the disease was also investigated, psychosocial comorbidities and quality of life, as well as treatment success. Data from September 2008 onwards corroborate significant associations between alexithymia and dermatological disease. Consistent with previous data, the prevalence of alexithymia in patients with skin disease (5–76.4%) is markedly higher than the prevalence of alexithymia in the general population (10%). In reference to vitiligo, a prevalence of clinically significant alexithymia of up to 65.4% in patients was reported [12]. A case-control study involving 52 patients found no significant difference in prevalence between patients and controls, but a cross-sectional study involving 30 patients did. In both studies, patients had significantly higher TAS-20 total scores than controls [14, 15]. Any study included in this review reported data on alexithymia after the treatment of diseases other than psoriasis and alopecia areata [12].

Regarding the physiological mechanisms linking alexithymia to dermatological disease, the "stress-alexithymia hypothesis" proposes that specific cognitive, behavioral, and physiological components of alexithymia may contribute to the pathogenesis of stress-related disorders, including dermatological diseases. According to this hypothesis, the combined effects of a lack of emotional awareness, as well as effective expression and verbalization (cognitive component), can lead to ineffective and/or maladaptive coping attempts (behavioral component). This, in turn, can lead to prolonged exposure to stress, which exacerbates the somatovisceral response (physiological component), thus increasing susceptibility to disease. In addition, it has been observed that the immune response of alexithymic subjects is similar to that of individuals exposed to chronic stress, with a higher production of glucocorticoids, a depressed cell-mediated immunity response, and an alteration of ratio Th1/Th2 (toward Th2 response). All of these findings are associated with cutaneous disease too [16, 17]. With regard to alexithymia and skin disease morbidity, perceived defects in physical appearance may develop significant emotional and social consequences, in particular, the experience of shame, stigmatization, social exclusion, and loneliness. Failure to discern psychological manifestations from physical symptoms can lead to additional inappropriate somatovisceral responses that further precipitate disease. Furthermore, this impaired emotional self-awareness and emotional regulation may also be related to impaired self-control, possibly worsening the duration and severity of the disease. So, beyond the high prevalence of alexithymia in dermatology patients, it may influence the development of psychosocial comorbidities and their treatment [12, 16, 17].

2.3 Anxiety and depression in vitiligo

Studies show that two-thirds of patients feel embarrassed and more than one-half report feeling socially anxious [18]. In one study of more than 600 patients, 59% of them reported an incident in the past three weeks in which their vitiligo had made them feel somehow bad [19]. More than a half of patients have been stared at, and 16% had overhead rude remarks, such as "Yuck, what´s wrong with him?" or "People like that should not go out in public" [20]. Moreover, when talking about the psychological aspects in vitiligo, Silvan M [21] reports that his patients described similar incidents, such as one man who told him how, when he holds the handrail on the subway, and the person next to him often moves his or her hand away. Many patients have also felt job discrimination [20].

Bearing all these experiences in mind, it is not difficult to understand the psychosocial impact of the disease and how it may impact mood and cause disorders, such as anxiety and depression.

A systematic search for observational studies that examined the prevalence of anxiety in vitiligo patients found 15 studies, including 1176 patients. The general prevalence of anxiety using random-effects models was 35.8%. A statistically significant difference in anxiety rates was found among female patients (47.32 vs. 42.4%) ($P = 0.03$). In addition, the pooled odds ratio among vitiligo and non-vitiligo patients did not indicate a statistical significance among patients coming from different continents, comparing African, European, Middle East, and South Asian countries [22].

On the other hand, a cross-sectional self-assessment questionnaire-based study conducted in Thailand, including 104 patients with vitiligo [23], showed the mean Dermatology Life Quality Index [24] score was 7.46, meaning a moderate impact on quality of life. Domains that had higher scores were those related to embarrassment, social activities, and clothing. Depression was evaluated using the Patient Health Questionnaire (PHQ-9) [25] and it showed scores equal to or above 9, which has been reported to be the optimal cutoff score for diagnosing major depression in the Thai population [26], in a 13.5% of patients. These patients showed higher scores for social activities, embarrassment, clothing, shopping, and homecare. Depression was considerably more frequent in patients with active vitiligo than in those with stable disease. Those patients with new appearing lesions were more likely to be depressed than those with no new macules [23]. Nevertheless, no differences were found when taking into account age, gender, educational level, skin phototype, or type of vitiligo [23]. Both questionnaire measures correlated well, meaning that higher levels of depression were found among patients with the worst quality of life and *vice versa* [23].

A recent study analyzes not only anxiety and depression but hopelessness [5] using the Beck´s Depression and Anxiety Inventory (BDI and BAI) [27, 28], the Beck´s Hopelessness Scale (BHS) [29], and the General Health Questionnaire (GHQ-28) [30] among 100 vitiligo patients and 100 healthy controls in an Iranian population. Anxiety and hopelessness levels were significantly higher in vitiligo patients than in control participants and this difference was more important among women with vitiligo.

All three variables had a positive and significant relationship with disease duration, but age had a negative relationship with all of them, so as younger they were, they felt worst.

It was also demonstrated that single patients were more anxious, hopeless, and depressive than those married. Patients living with their couples were only more anxious and hopeless than healthy controls.

Vitiligo patients, women in special, showed the worst general health in this study [5].

We can also consider the role of stress, along with anxiety and depression. A cross-sectional study includes 50 vitiligo patients and 50 matched healthy controls [4] in which all patients were assessed by the Depression Anxiety Stress Scale (DASS) [31] to determine the severity of these three aspects and, Dermatology Life Quality Index (DLQI) [24] only in vitiligo patients, to evaluate the impact of the disease on daily life [4]; disease activity was measured using Vitiligo Area and Severity Index [32], and showed that the prevalence of stress was 76%, anxiety 78%, and depression 80% among vitiligo patients, and the difference was statistically significant between patients and controls. They also found that stress, anxiety, and depression were higher among women ($P < 0.05$). The degree of the disease implies more anxiety and depression ($p > 0.05$). The familiar history of vitiligo had a positive relationship with depression. Nevertheless, this study failed to demonstrate any statistically significant correlation with age, marital status, type of work, type of vitiligo, site of the lesions, and type of therapy with stress, anxiety, or depression. It is also interesting that they found a positive correlation between stress and feelings of embarrassment from vitiligo and clothes choice [4]. They feel embarrassed, and try to hide the lesions with clothes and it means more stress.

Another recent study conducted in Egypt [33] collected 100 patients with vitiligo that were subjected to clinical examination and disease activity was measured with VASI; they were compared with 50 healthy controls and assessed for quality of life with the DLQI and for anxiety and depression with the Hamilton Anxiety Rating Scale (HARS) [34, 35]. This tool rates depression by probing mood, feelings of guilt, suicide ideation, insomnia, agitation or retardation, weight loss, and somatic symptoms. They found higher scores on DLQI, showing worst levels of quality of life among patients ($P<0.001$), and also significant differences in the Hamilton Anxiety and Depression Score than the control group. A significant positive correlation was found between VASI score and extension of the disease, in special those with exposed areas of skin affected, with DLQI and HARS. Patients with a progressive course of the disease showed the worst quality of life. Female patients also showed higher levels of impairment. Although not significant, patients with lower skin phototypes showed lower levels of depression and better quality of life [33].

As stated above, alexithymic people have a lower ability to deal with difficult life events. As anxiety and depression, alexithymia might be a triggering factor for diseases [36, 37]. Namdar ND and Kurtoglu Y [38] conducted a study, including 50 vitiligo patients and 70 healthy controls, matched in age and sex and investigated anxiety, depression, and alexithymia among them. They grouped patients as generalized and localized vitiligo according to their clinical involvement. Depression was assessed with the Beck Depression Inventory [35], anxiety with the Beck Anxiety Inventory [28], and alexithymia using the Toronto Alexithymia Scale with 20 items, TAS-20 [39, 40]. Anxiety and depression levels were higher in vitiligo patients than in healthy control individuals ($P = 0.000$, $P = 0.009$ respectively), but no differences between alexithymia scores ($P = 0.103$). No correlation could be found between psychiatric scale scores and disease duration, age or gender of patients, or educational levels. Nevertheless, alexithymia levels correlated positively with anxiety and depression levels in vitiligo patients [38]. So, when psychosocial impairment is evident, feelings might be more difficult to recognize and show to patients, and these facts do not help them at all.

In 2009 ESDAP Congress, we report a case-control study that included 100 patients with vitiligo who attended our outpatient clinics between January and August, and 100 control subjects without clinical history of vitiligo. The aim was to analyze the prevalence of depression and/or anxiety in patients with vitiligo. All the patients were older than 16 years old. Both groups were matched in age and sex. They were included consecutively, using the Spanish version of the Hospital Anxiety and Depression Scale (HADS) [41]. The statistical analysis was performed with the

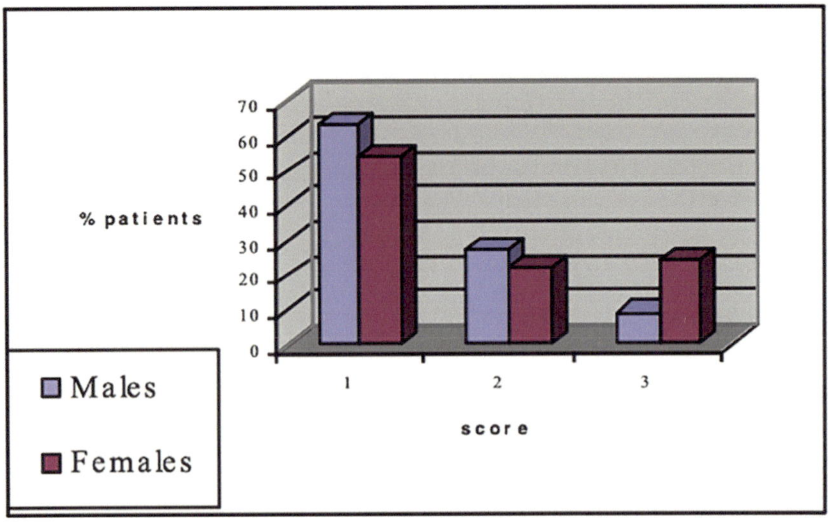

Figure 3.
Anxiety and probably anxiety cases distributed by gender.

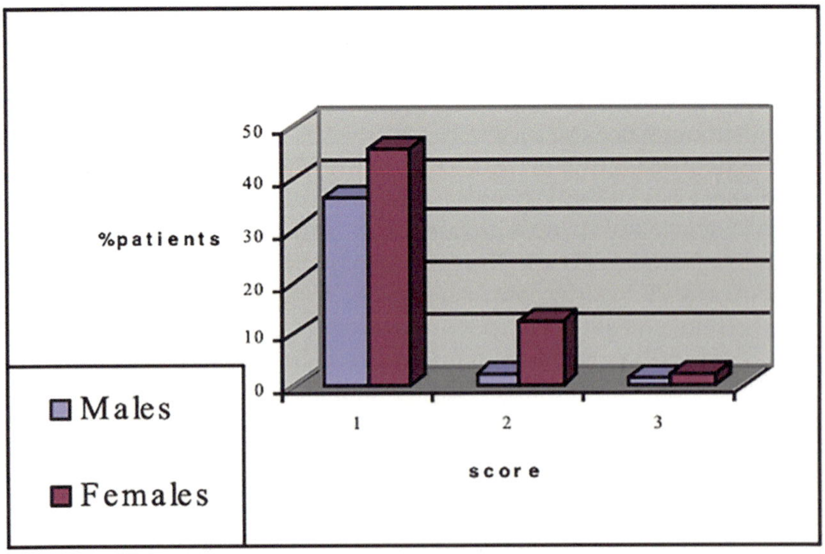

Figure 4.
Depression and probably depression cases distributed by gender.

SPSS program version 17.0. For the depression subscale, 3 patients had a score of 11 or higher (3.6%), 12 between 8 and 10 (14.5%), and 68 of 7 or lower (81.9%). For anxiety, 15 had a score of 11 or higher (18.1%), 20 between 8 and 10 (24.1%), and 48 of 7 or lower (57.8%). Anxiety was more frequent in women (24% in women vs. 9.1% in men) (**Figure 3**). Women also showed more cases (4% vs. 3%) and probable cases (20% vs. 6.1%) of depression (**Figure 4**). However, no significant differences were found between the sexes for anxiety or depression ($p=0.224$ and $p=0.196$). The prevalence of anxiety between age groups showed significant differences ($p=0.022$, $p<0.05$). In the analysis, differences were observed between patients aged 37–46 years and those over 66, who presented the highest and lowest frequency of cases, respectively. Higher levels of anxiety correlate with higher levels of depression ($Rho=0.609$, $p<0.0001$) [42].

3. Psychological approach

Patients with vitiligo usually feel socially isolated and with limitations in their daily life and that's why they usually present depressive and anxious symptomatology. Therefore, it is very important that vitiligo treatment includes a complete psychological intervention. Moreover, data show that a multidisciplinary treatment in this type of patient can slow down the progression of vitiligo and even reduce the size of affected areas. It is usually patients with psychological deficits and strong emotional vulnerability and this is why it's hard to find the right treatment. Taking this into account, it is crucial to take medical and psychological treatment simultaneously [21].

In view of the above, it would be accurate to give some surveys to the patients in order to have a qualitative and quantitative description of their psychological state. The surveys that we can use are Toronto Alexithymia Scale (TAS-20), Dermatology Life Quality Index (DLQI), and Beck Depression Inventory (BDI-II).

3.1 Toronto Alexithymia Scale (TAS-20)

This scale (**Figure 5**) was developed by Bagby, Parker and Taylor in 1994 [40] from former versions with 26 and 23 questions.

The TAS-20 is based on three factors:

- Evaluation of difficulty in identification of feelings and distinguishing them from physiological sensations that go with emotional activity (factor 1).
- Difficulty in describing feelings (factor 2).
- Thought focused on the external (factor 3).

It is a self-report with 20 questions, with a Likert-type scale of 5 points that show from "total agree" to "total disagree" with each of the statements [39].

3.2 Dermatology Life Quality Index (DLQI)

The DLQI survey (**Figure 6**) was developed in the U. K by AY Finlay and GK Khan in 1994 [24]. This instrument is simple, sensitive, and compact. It is made of 10 questions referred to in the last seven days. It presents a Likert-type scale with four

Toronto Alexithymia Scale
I have feelings that I can't quite identify I often don't know why I am angry It is difficult for me to find the right words for my feelings I am often puzzled by sensations in my body I am often confused about what emotion I am feeling I have physical sensations that even doctors don't understand I find it hard to describe how I feel about people I don't know what's going on inside me When I'm upset, I don't know if I'm sad, frightened, or angry I wish I were not so shy I'm able to describe my feelings easily When I cry I always know why
I spend much time daydreaming whenever I have nothing else to do I daydream rarely I use my imagination a great deal I often daydream about the future Daydreaming is a waste of time
I prefer to analyze problems rather than just describe them One should look for deeper explanations I like to let people know where I stand on things It's not enough for me that something gets the job done; I need to know why and how it works People tell me to describe my feelings more
Knowing the answers to problems is more important than knowing the reasons for the answers I prefer to just let things happen rather than to understand why they turned out that way Being in touch with emotions is essential I seem to make friends as easily as others do

Figure 5.
Toronto Alexithymia Scale.

possible answers: «not at all», «a little», «a lot» o «very much», with respective 0, 1, 2, and 3 punctuation, also having the possibility «not relevant». The health domains included in DLQI are as follows:

- Symptoms and perceptions (questions 1, 2).
- Daily activities (3, 4).
- Leisure (5, 6).
- Work/study (7).

- Interpersonal relationships, including sexuality (8, 9).

- Treatment (10).

The total punctuation will give us a global value from 0–30. Such punctuation could be presented as the percentage of the impact of skin affection on the patient's life quality. The more punctuation, the more impact on life quality related to patient's health (HRQOL) [43].

DERMATOLOGY LIFE QUALITY INDEX (DLQI)

Hospital No: .... **Date:** ....

Name: .... **Score:** ....

Address: .... **Diagnosis:** ....

....

The aim of this questionnaire is to measure how much your skin problem has affected your life OVER THE LAST WEEK. Please tick (✓) one box for each question.

1.	Over the last week, how **itchy**, **sore**, **painful** or **stinging** has your skin been?	Very much A lot A little Not at all	☐ ☐ ☐ ☐	
2.	Over the last week, how **embarrassed** or **self conscious** have you been because of your skin?	Very much A lot A little Not at all	☐ ☐ ☐ ☐	
3.	Over the last week, how much has your skin interfered with you going **shopping** or looking after your **home** or **garden**?	Very much A lot A little Not at all	☐ ☐ ☐ ☐	Not relevant ☐
4.	Over the last week, how much has your skin influenced the **clothes** you wear?	Very much A lot A little Not at all	☐ ☐ ☐ ☐	Not relevant ☐
5.	Over the last week, how much has your skin affected any **social** or **leisure** activities?	Very much A lot A little Not at all	☐ ☐ ☐ ☐	Not relevant ☐
6.	Over the last week, how much has your skin made it difficult for you to do any **sport**?	Very much A lot A little Not at all	☐ ☐ ☐ ☐	Not relevant ☐
7.	Over the last week, has your skin prevented you from **working** or **studying**?	Yes No	☐ ☐	Not relevant ☐
	If "No", over the last week how much has your skin been a problem at **work** or **studying**?	A lot A little Not at all	☐ ☐ ☐	
8.	Over the last week, how much has your skin created problems with your **partner** or any of your **close friends** or **relatives**?	Very much A lot A little Not at all	☐ ☐ ☐ ☐	Not relevant ☐
9.	Over the last week, how much has your skin caused any **sexual difficulties**?	Very much A lot A little Not at all	☐ ☐ ☐ ☐	Not relevant ☐
10.	Over the last week, how much of a problem has the **treatment** for your skin been, for example by making your home messy, or by taking up time?	Very much A lot A little Not at all	☐ ☐ ☐ ☐	Not relevant ☐

Please check you have answered EVERY question. Thank you.

Figure 6.
Dermatology Life Quality Index.

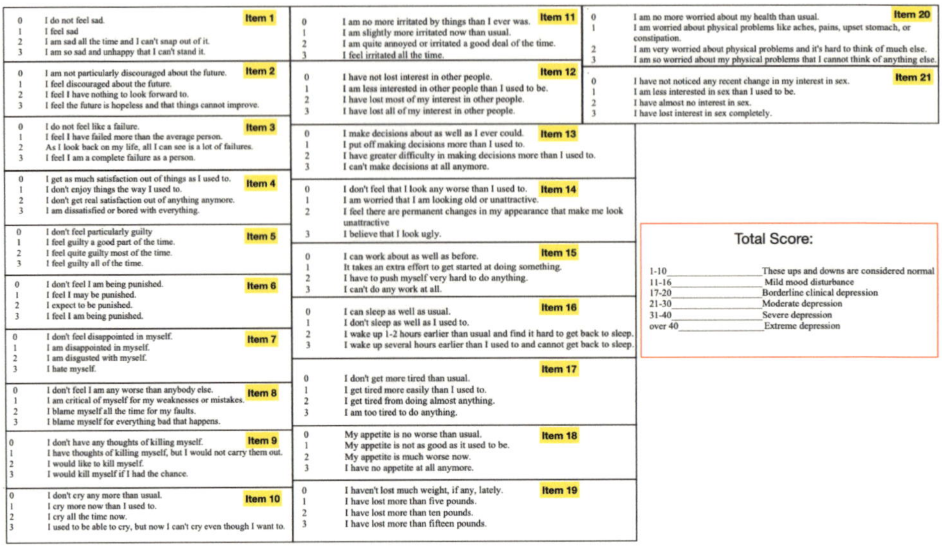

Item 1
0 I do not feel sad.
1 I feel sad
2 I am sad all the time and I can't snap out of it.
3 I am so sad and unhappy that I can't stand it.

Item 2
0 I am not particularly discouraged about the future.
1 I feel discouraged about the future.
2 I feel I have nothing to look forward to.
3 I feel the future is hopeless and that things cannot improve.

Item 3
0 I do not feel like a failure.
1 I feel I have failed more than the average person.
2 As I look back on my life, all I can see is a lot of failures.
3 I feel I am a complete failure as a person.

Item 4
0 I get as much satisfaction out of things as I used to.
1 I don't enjoy things the way I used to.
2 I don't get real satisfaction out of anything anymore.
3 I am dissatisfied or bored with everything.

Item 5
0 I don't feel particularly guilty
1 I feel guilty a good part of the time.
2 I feel quite guilty most of the time.
3 I feel guilty all of the time.

Item 6
0 I don't feel I am being punished.
1 I feel I may be punished.
2 I expect to be punished.
3 I feel I am being punished.

Item 7
0 I don't feel disappointed in myself.
1 I am disappointed in myself.
2 I am disgusted with myself.
3 I hate myself.

Item 8
0 I don't feel I am any worse than anybody else.
1 I am critical of myself for my weaknesses or mistakes.
2 I blame myself all the time for my faults.
3 I blame myself for everything bad that happens.

Item 9
0 I don't have any thoughts of killing myself.
1 I have thoughts of killing myself, but I would not carry them out.
2 I would like to kill myself.
3 I would kill myself if I had the chance.

Item 10
0 I don't cry any more than usual.
1 I cry more now than I used to.
2 I cry all the time now.
3 I used to be able to cry, but now I can't cry even though I want to.

Item 11
0 I am no more irritated by things than I ever was.
1 I am slightly more irritated now than usual.
2 I am quite annoyed or irritated a good deal of the time.
3 I feel irritated all the time.

Item 12
0 I have not lost interest in other people.
1 I am less interested in other people than I used to be.
2 I have lost most of my interest in other people.
3 I have lost all of my interest in other people.

Item 13
0 I make decisions about as well as I ever could.
1 I put off making decisions more than I used to.
2 I have greater difficulty in making decisions more than I used to.
3 I can't make decisions at all anymore.

Item 14
0 I don't feel that I look any worse than I used to.
1 I am worried that I am looking old or unattractive.
2 I feel there are permanent changes in my appearance that make me look unattractive
3 I believe that I look ugly.

Item 15
0 I can work about as well as before.
1 It takes an extra effort to get started at doing something.
2 I have to push myself very hard to do anything.
3 I can't do any work at all.

Item 16
0 I can sleep as well as usual.
1 I don't sleep as well as I used to.
2 I wake up 1-2 hours earlier than usual and find it hard to get back to sleep.
3 I wake up several hours earlier than I used to and cannot get back to sleep.

Item 17
0 I don't get more tired than usual.
1 I get tired more easily than I used to.
2 I get tired from doing almost anything.
3 I am too tired to do anything.

Item 18
0 My appetite is no worse than usual.
1 My appetite is not as good as it used to be.
2 My appetite is much worse now.
3 I have no appetite at all anymore.

Item 19
0 I haven't lost much weight, if any, lately.
1 I have lost more than five pounds.
2 I have lost more than ten pounds.
3 I have lost more than fifteen pounds.

Item 20
0 I am no more worried about my health than usual.
1 I am worried about physical problems like aches, pains, upset stomach, or constipation.
2 I am very worried about physical problems and it's hard to think of much else.
3 I am so worried about my physical problems that I cannot think of anything else.

Item 21
0 I have not noticed any recent change in my interest in sex.
1 I am less interested in sex than I used to be.
2 I have almost no interest in sex.
3 I have lost interest in sex completely.

Total Score:

1-10	These ups and downs are considered normal
11-16	Mild mood disturbance
17-20	Borderline clinical depression
21-30	Moderate depression
31-40	Severe depression
over 40	Extreme depression

Figure 7.
Beck Depression Inventory.

3.3 Beck Depression Inventory (BDI-II)

The original version of the Beck Depression Inventory was published in 1961 by Beck, Ward, Mendelson, and Erbaugh [9] and updated in 1996 by Aaron T. Beck, Robert A. Steer and Gregory K. Brown (BDI-II). It is a self-report made up of 21 Likert-type items. Its items do not arise from any specific theory about depression but describe the most frequent clinical symptoms of patients with depression, such as sadness, crying, loss of pleasure, failure and guilt feelings, suicide thoughts or desire, and pessimism [44].

As previously mentioned, the BDI-II versión (**Figure 7**) was published in 1996, while in 2011, Jesús Sanz and Carmelo Vázquez, published the Spanish adaptation of this test [45].

This inventory is of great relevance and that is why it is considered the fifth most used test by Spanish psychologists [46].

4. Psychological treatment

4.1 Depression

The cognitive therapy (CT) developed by Aaron T Beck in the late 50s is the most accurate procedure to treat depression since it's specifically designed to work on this construct.

The CT gives us a complete concept of depression because it presents:

- A theory.
- A diagnostic evaluation.
- A therapeutic procedure.

With this theory, depression is explained by the existence of negative thoughts about oneself, about the world, and/or the future. This is due to depressive factors and failure in processing information.

This type of psychological treatment is very organized and consists of 15–25 sessions, including continuation and termination sessions. The CT is conceived from a psychoeducational point of view, since it tries to modify cognitions and behaviors. That is why it is also named as cognitive-behavioral therapy (CBT) [47].

The main features of this theory are the following:

- It emphasizes the relationship between cognitions, behavior, and emotions.
- It must be formulated individually in order to establish the therapeutic goals and the treatment to be followed.
- A good therapeutic relationship is key to achieve change.
- The patients will obtain a new way to understand their problems.
- It is focused on the current factors that sustain the problem.
- It needs active collaboration between therapist and patient.
- The patients will get the resources and skills required to manage their problems autonomously.
- It's short (usually less than 30 sessions).
- The activities between sessions are very important for the treatment.
- It uses many cognitive and behavioral techniques and other approaches, such as full consciousness or mindfulness [48]

4.2 Anxiety

It is very important to know the existing differences between the different anxiety disorders and to know the diagnostic criteria of each one of them in order to take the right treatment in vitiligo patients. Otherwise, in many cases, in primary care medicine, anxiety disorders are not diagnosed. And this is why it is very important to detect and work on them.

In order to make an appropriate treatment, we must know the three components of anxiety, which are subjective fear, physiological activation, and avoiding behavior. These three components do not always change in the same way. So, the treatment will be aimed at that anxiety component that is affecting the patient. The effective physiological intervention trains an individual to reduce physiological activation through biofeedback and with several relaxing skills. Each method leads to self-calm of the body and reduction in physiology of stress and alert, so the patient will manage subjective fear. Cognitive therapy teaches the patients to modify fearful thoughts and redirect their attention far from fears, and self-training to overcome fearful experiences. With all the above, a full recovery needs a change in the cognitive-affective area, physiology activation, and behavioral avoidance [49].

4.3 Alexthymia

Over the years, changes have been proposed in order to conceptualize and measure alexithymia. This psychological feature has been related to several disorders. In general, psychotherapy seems to be useful to patients with alexithymia. There are several aspects that will help the patient to build a consistent narrative and explore the emotional dimensions. These aspects are the development of vocabulary in emotions, the learning of reading the emotions of others, and the relation between alexithymia and early life experiences. With this, we develop social and emotional skills. Interventions could be made individually or in groups. Another important aspect of the therapeutic process in patients with alexithymia is the empathy of the therapist. This allows the understanding of others, their goals, intentions and feelings, makes exploration easier, promotes the opening to new experiences and a curious behavior toward emotional experiences, and at the same time allows the deconstruction of assumptions and values [50].

Several neurobiological studies performed so far suggest that people who present alexithymia usually have a deficit in emotion recognition. Therefore, effective treatments for alexithymia include the training of skills in the domain of emotion recognition. It has been proven that the interventions based on smartphones (SBI), which offer training in skills, are great complements of psychological treatments. In 2019, a pilot study with 29 subjects with high levels of alexithymia were randomly assigned to an intervention group (SBI group) or a control group. Participants assigned to SBI group received a psychoeducation session and 14 days of training with the app *alexitimia mindtastic* (*MT-ALEX*) and the control group only received the psychoeducation session. MT-ALEX includes 14 emotion-specific workouts for training inter- and intraindividual recognition of seven basic emotions: fear, anger, disgust, sadness, joy, pride, and surprise. The results showed higher rates of emotion recognition skills by the SBI group. By this way, the SBI could improve emotion recognition skills in patients with alexithymia [51].

5. Conclusions

Vitiligo is one of the most psychologically devastating diseases in dermatology. Although the contrast of vitiligo lesions is more visible in racial/ethnic groups with darker skin, all vitiligo patients experience some degree of emotional disturbance caused by the disease. Therefore, health professionals should be aware that patients suffer from a significant psychosocial burden, which suggests that vitiligo treatment will always be necessary, not only for esthetic purposes. It is very important to recognize and assess the psychological and social problems of this disease to improve quality of life and treatment results.

In addition, an added factor is the high prevalence of alexithymia in these patients, as this may influence the development of other psychosocial comorbidities and their treatment. It is likely that early recognition and management of the alexithymia may improve dermatological care, mitigate psychological comorbidities, improve quality of life, improve self-management, get stronger patient-physician relationships, and reduce inappropriate use of drugs and health resources. More randomized clinical trials should be conducted to investigate the usefulness of therapeutic approaches targeting alexithymia to improve disease outcomes and quality of life for patients.

In conclusion, psychodermatology is a necessary subspecialty in our daily dermatological practice, especially in patients with vitiligo.

Acknowledgements

Acknowledgments go to CHUC dermatology department, especially Dr. Noda Cabrera, Dra. Marina Rodríguez y Dra. Patricia Contreras.

Acknowledgments go to Luis Trujillo Brito, Dermamedicin's Director, and Manager.

Conflict of interest

The authors declare no conflict of interest.

Author details

Nayra Merino[1,2]*, Mónica Fumero[1,2], Maria Eugenia Gaviño[1,2] and Marta García-Bustinduy[1,2]

1 Dermamedicin Clinics, Santa Cruz de Tenerife, Spain

2 Hospital Universitario de. Canarias, La Laguna, Spain

*Address all correspondence to: nayra.merino@dermamedicin.com

References

[1] Ezzedine K, Eleftheriadou V, Jones H, Bibeau K, Kuo FI, Sturm D, et al. Psychosocial effects of Vitiligo: A systematic literature review. American Journal of Clinical Dermatology. 2021;**22**(6):757-774

[2] Mattoo SK, Handa S, Kaur I, Gupta N, Malhotra R. Psychiatric morbidity in vitiligo: Prevalence and correlates in India. Journal of the European Academy of Dermatology and Venereology. 2002;**16**(6):573-578

[3] Grimes PE, Miller MM. Vitiligo: Patient stories, self-esteem, and the psychological burden of disease. International Journal of Women's Dermatology. 2018;**4**(1):32-37

[4] Nasser MA, Raggi SM, Abdelfatah ZA, et al. Stress, anxiety, and depression in patients with vitiligo. Middle East Current Psychiatry. 2021;**28**:63

[5] Hamidizadeh N, Ranjbar S, Ghanizadeh A, et al. Evaluating prevalence of depression, anxiety and hopelessness in patients with Vitiligo on an Iranian population. Health and Quality of Life Outcomes. 2020;**18**:20

[6] Grimes P. Aesthetics and Cosmetic Surgery for Darker Skin Types. New York: Lippincott; 2008

[7] Do Bú EA, Alexandre MES, Scardua A, Araújo CRF. Vitiligo as a psychosocial disease: Apprehensions of patients imprinted by the white. Interface (Botucatu). 2018;**22**(65):481-491

[8] Silverberg JI, Silverberg NB. Association between vitiligo extent and distribution and quality-of-life impairment. JAMA Dermatology. 2013;**149**(2):159-164

[9] Elbuluk N, Ezzedine K. Quality of life, burden of disease, co-morbidities, and systemic effects in vitiligo patients. Dermatologic Clinics. 2017;**35**(2):117-128

[10] Linthorst Homan MW, De Korte J, Grootenhuis MA, Bos JD, Sprangers MA, Van Der Veen JP. Impact of childhood vitiligo on adult life. The British Journal of Dermatology. 2008;**159**(4):915-920

[11] Namdar ND, Kurtoglu Y. Alexithymia, anxiety, and depression in patients with vitiligo. Annals of Medical Research. 2021;**28**(4):663-667

[12] Holmes A, Marella P, Rodriguez C, Donald Glass II, Goerlich KS. Alexithymia and cutaneous disease morbidity: A systematic review. Dermatology. May 30, 2022:1-10

[13] Willemsen R, Roseeuw D, Vanderlinden J. Alexithymia and dermatology: The state of the art. International Journal of Dermatology. 2008;**47**(9):903-910

[14] Maghami Z, Sepaskhah M, Sarani EM, Bagheri Z, Maghami M. Alexithymia in vitiligo patients: A case-control study. Iranian Journal of Dermatology. 2018;**21**:138-141

[15] Dehghani F, Dehghani F, Kafaie P. Alexithymia in different dermato- logic patients. Asian Journal of Psychiatry. 2017;**25**:42-45

[16] Guilbaud O, Corcos M, Hjalmarsson L, Loas G, Jeammet P. Is there a psychoneuroimmu- nological pathway between alexithymia and immunity? Immune and physiological

corre- lates of alexithymia. Biomedicine & Pharmacotherapy. 2003;**57**(7):292-295

[17] Guilbaud O, Curt F, Perrin C, Chaouat G, Berthoz S, Dugré-Le Bigre C, et al. Decreased immune response in alexithymic women: A cross-sectional study. Biomedicine & Pharmacotherapy. 2009;**63**(4):297-230

[18] Porter J, Beuf AH, Nordlund JJ, Lerner AB. Psychological reaction to chronic skin disorders: A study of patients with vitiligo. General Hospital Psychiatry. 1979;**112**:73-77

[19] Kent G, Abadie M. Psychologic effects of vitiligo: A critical incident analysis. Journal of the American Academy of Dermatology. 1996;**35**:895-898

[20] Porter JR, Beuf AH, Lemer A, Nordlund JJ. Psycholosocial effect of vitiligo: A comparison of vitiligo patients with "normal" control subjects, with psoriasis patients and with patients with other pigmentary disorders. Journal of the American Academy of Dermatology. 1986;**15**:220-224

[21] Silvan M. The psychological factors of vitiligo. Cutis. 2004;**73**:163-167

[22] Dussainova A, Kassym L, Akhmetova A, Glushkova N, Sabirov U, Adilgonzhina S, et al. Vitiligo and anxiety: A systematic review and meta-analysis. PLoS One. 2020;**15**:e024

[23] Silpa-archa N, Pruksaea C, Angkoolpakdeekul N, Chaiyabutr C, Kulthanan K, Ratta-apa W, et al. Relationship between depression and quality of life among vitiligo patients: A self-assessment Quesionnaire-based study. Clinical, Cosmetic and Investigational Dermatology. 2020;**13**:511-520

[24] Finlay AI, Khan GK. Dermatology Life Quality Index (DLQI)-a simple practical measure for routine clinical use. Clinical and Experimental Dermatology. 1994;**19**:210-216

[25] Kroenke K, Spitzer RL, Williams JB. The PHQ-9: Validity of a brief depression severity measure. Journal of General Internal Medicine. 2001;**16**:606-613

[26] Lotrakul M, Sumrithe S, Saipanish R. Reliability and validity of the Thai version of the PHQ-9. BMC Psychiatry. 2008;**8**:46

[27] Beck AT, Ward CH, Mendelson M, Mock J, Erbaugh J. An inventory for measuring depression. Archives of General Psychiatry. 1961;**4**:561-571

[28] Beck AT, Epstein N, Brown G, Steer RA. An inventory for measuring clinical anxiety: Psychometric properties. Journal of Consulting and Clinical Psychology. 1988;**56**:893-897

[29] Beck AT, Weissman A, Lester D, Trexler L. The measurement of pessimism: The hopelessness scale. Journal of Consulting and Clinical Psychology. 1974;**42**:861-865

[30] Goldberg DP, Hiller VF. A scaled version of the general health questionnaire. Psychological Medicine. 1979;**9**:39-45

[31] Lovibond SH, Lovibond PF. Manual for the Depression Anxiety & Stress Scales. Sydney: Psychology Foundation; 1995

[32] Hamzavi I, Jain H, McLean D, Shapiro J, Zeng H, Lui H. Paramedic model of narrow band UVB phototherapy for vitiligo using a novel quantitative tool: The Vitiligo Area Scoring Index. Archives of Dermatology. 2004;**140**:677-682

[33] Abdelmaguid EM, Khalifa H, Salah MM, Sayed DS. Assessment of depression and anxiety in relation to quality of life in patients with vitiligo. Egyptian Journal of Dermatology and Venereology. 2020;**40**:99-105

[34] Hamilton M. Arating scale for depression. Journal of Neurology. 1960;**23**:42-56

[35] Porter E, Chambless DL, McCArthy KS, DeRubels RJ, Sharpless BA, Barrett MS, et al. Psychomedic properties of the reconstructed Hamilton depression and anxiety scales. The Journal of Nervous and Mental Diseases. 2017;**205**:656-660

[36] Sifneos PE. Alexithymia and its relationship to hemispheric specialization, affect, and creativity. The Psychiatric Clinics of North America. 1988;**11**:287-292

[37] Picardi A, Pasquini P, Cattaruzza MS, et al. Stressful life events, social support, attachment security and alexithymiain vitiligo. A case-control studio. Psychotherapy Psychosomatics. 2003;**72**:150-158

[38] Namdar ND, Kurtoglu Y. Alexithymia, axiety, and depression in patients with vitiligo. Annals of Medical Research. 2021;**29**:663-667

[39] Bagby RM, Parker JD, Taylor GJ. The twenty-item Toronto Alexithymia Scale-I. Item selection and cross-validation of the factor structure. Journal of Psychosomatic Research. 1994;**38**:23-32

[40] Bagby RM, Parker JDA, Taylor GJ. The Twenty-item Toronto Alexithymia Scale-II. Convergent, discriminant, and concurrent validity. Journal of Psychosomatic Research. 1994;**38**:33-40

[41] Ibáñez E, y Caro I. La escala Hospitalaria de ansiedad y depresión. Su utilidad práctica en Psicología de la Salud. Boletín de Psicología. 1992;**36**:43-69

[42] Paz N, Rodríguez-Martín M, Noda Cabrera A, García Bustínduy M. Anxiety and depression in vitiligo outpatients. A case-control study. Acta Dermato-Venereologica. 2009;**89**:551-592

[43] De Tiedra AG, Mercadal J, Badía X, Mascaró JM, Herdamn M, Lozano R. Transcultural adaptation of the questionnaire Dermatology Life Quality Index (DLQI): El Índice de Calidad de Vida en Dermatología. Actas Dermo-Sifiliográficas. 1998;**89**(12):692-700

[44] Beck AT, Steer RA, Brown GK. BDI-II. Beck Depression Inventory. San Antonio, TX: The Psychological Corporation; 1996

[45] Sanz J. Adaptación española del Inventario para la Depresión de Beck-II (BDI-II): 2. Propiedades psicométricas en población general. Clínica y Salud. 2003;**14**(3):249-280. https://www.redalyc.org/articulo.oa?id=180617972001

[46] Muñiz J, Fernández-Hermida JR. La opinión de los psicólogos españoles sobre el uso de los test. Papeles del Psicólogo. 2010;**31**:108-121

[47] Pérez M, García JM. Tratamientos psciológicos eficaces para la depresión. Psicothema. 2001;**13**(3):493-510

[48] Badós A. Terapia cognitiva de Beck. In: En Labrador FJ, editor. Técnicas de modificación de conducta. España: Pirámide; 2011. pp. 517-533

[49] Moss D. Psychological perspectives: Anxiety disorders identification and intervention. In: Horwitz, editor.

Communication Apprehension: Origins and Management. 1st ed. Australia: Singular/Thompson Learning; 2002

[50] Nunes da Silva A. Developing emotional skills and the therapeutic alliance in clients with alexithymia: Intervention guidelines. Psychopathology. 2021;**54**:282-290. DOI: 10.1159/000519786

[51] Lukas CA, Trevisi Fuentes H, Berking M. Smartphone-based emotion recognition skills training for alexithymia—A randomized controlled pilot study. Internet Interventions. 2019;**17**:100250

Section 3

Medications and Pigmentation Disorders

Chapter 5

Skin Depigmenting Agents: Where Do We Stand?

Behrooz Kasraee

Abstract

Skin hyperpigmentary disorders are frequent and psychologically disturbing conditions for patients. Skin depigmenting agents have been widely used for the treatment of such disorders. The most efficacious depigmenting agents, such as hydroquinone and the Kligman's formula, are associated with long-term side effects, and safer skin depigmenting agents, such as kojic acid, arbutin, and niacinamide, might suffer from a significantly lower depigmenting efficacy. Therefore, there is still a need for safe and simultaneously efficacious skin depigmenting compounds. Tranexamic acid and cysteamine are two new and interesting molecules that seem to fulfill the majority of the needed characteristics of an acceptable skin depigmenting agent. In this chapter, a review of most important molecules as well as their side effects will be provided with a focus on the newest skin depigmenting molecules recently emerged into the armamentarium of hyperpigmentation treatments.

Keywords: hyperpigmentation, depigmenting molecules, melanogenesis, melanin

1. Introduction

As dermatologists, we often find ourselves confronted with patients suffering from hyperpigmentation disorders such as, post-inflammatory hyperpigmentation (PIH), melasma, solar lentigines as well as facial dyschromia. What we see as dark spots or patches on the skin is the result of altered melanin production and/or melanocyte density. Focal hyperpigmentation typically occurs after skin injury or other causes of inflammation including acne vulgaris and eczema. Chronic exposure to UV light also represents a risk factor for the development of skin hyperpigmentation as well as premature aging due to the oxidative stress and cellular damage caused by UVA and UVB rays. These conditions generally do not impact health of the patients; however, as they may significantly affect their appearance, they can be psychologically disturbing and have an impact on patient's quality of life. According to a recent study, patients with pigmentary disorders have a high prevalence of psychological distress, including stress, anxiety, and depression [1]. Therefore, it is of utmost importance for patients' psychological well-being to provide them with efficacious and safe treatments for short- as well as long-term use. Maintenance therapy is especially important in hyperpigmentation disorders such as melasma, which has a high recurrence rate. However, the most effective depigmenting agents that are currently available in the armamentarium of dermatologists often take long to show results, have poor patient compliance, and/or do not have a safety profile that allow long-term use due to the risk of causing unwanted side effects.

In this chapter, the most efficacious topical, oral, and injectable depigmenting agents for treating hyperpigmentation will be discussed, and special attention will be given to the most recent and promising ones.

2. Skin depigmenting agents throughout history

Skin whitening is an ancient practice with a long and complex history. In ancient Greece, women painted their faces with white lead to achieve a lighter and unblemished skin tone as at that time pale skin was a sign of beauty and prestige [2]. Ancient Egyptians, like other Mediterranean populations, used to lighten their skin as well. Corroborating this was the uncovering of a 3500-year-old mummy head in the area of the Theban necropolis that exhibited pathological signs typical of exogenous ochronosis, an inflammatory skin condition, which is currently linked to the long-term and unsupervised application of creams containing the depigmenting agent hydroquinone [3]. In ancient Rome, people used a mixture of vinegar and white lead (called cerussa, the lead sugar) with the purpose of whitening their faces. Another widely used skin lightening ingredient was mercury. Creams and ointments containing mercury have been used for centuries to treat infections as well as inflammatory skin diseases and more recently as topical skin whiteners or "freckle removers" [4]. Inorganic mercury compounds are absorbed through the skin and cause depigmentation by competing with copper and resulting in an inactivation of tyrosinase, the enzyme responsible for melanin synthesis. After World War II, the toxic effects of mercury and lead became more evident. Cases of nephrotic syndrome as well as gastrointestinal and neurotoxicity were associated to the use of mercury-containing skin lightening products [5]. Finally, in 1973, the FDA banned the use of mercury in cosmetics [6]. Mercury was therefore replaced by other active ingredients, i.e., hydroquinone, which became the gold standard depigmenting agent for the treatment of hyperpigmentation. Hydroquinone also encountered safety concerns in recent years due to its potential mutagenic effect and was banned in several countries. This let dermatologists and patients with few options for the treatment of hyperpigmentary disorders. Oral and injectable tranexamic acid and topical cysteamine entered into the scope of effective depigmenting options, and much research has been done on these two promising molecules in recent years.

2.1 Topical treatments

The first-line treatment for hyperpigmentation involves topical application of formulations incorporating depigmenting agents. If such options do not prove to be efficacious in the patient, more invasive treatments such as microneedling, mesotherapy, microdermabrasion, chemical peels, or laser are often performed. These however might be associated with post-inflammatory hyperpigmentation especially in higher phototypes. On the other hand, these methods are rather invasive and costly, and a long-term maintenance treatment is usually not acceptable by the patients. Oral administration of drugs, e.g., tranexamic acid (TXA), is usually considered as last therapeutic option. Although TXA treatment is very effective, the risk of life-threatening side effects such as thrombus formation causes it to be hardly acceptable for the treatment of "cosmetic" problems. The optimal treatment for hyperpigmentary disorders would thus be a topical treatment employable by patients at home and not only effective, but also safe enough to be used long term as the maintenance therapy. The most well-known topical depigmenting molecules will be discussed in the next sections. Their efficacy as well as safety profile for long-term use will be addressed, and the most appropriate topical depigmenting agent available today will be discussed in more detail.

2.1.1 Hydroquinone and its derivatives

Hydroquinone (HQ) is a biphenol. Its widespread application in human and industrial activities made hydroquinone a ubiquitous molecule in the environment. In 1936, Oettel reported that black-haired cats turned gray when fed with HQ over a period of 6–8 weeks, and after stopping the treatment, the hair became repigmented as quick [7]. This finding was confirmed a few years later by Martin and Ansbacher [8].

In 1939, Oliver et al. published about an antioxidant (monobenzylether of hydroquinone) used in rubber gloves to reduce their deterioration, which was responsible for depigmentation of the skin of workers wearing the gloves [9]. In 1941, Peck and Sobotka found out that oral administration monobenzylether of hydroquinone to guinea pigs did not result in any depigmentation. However, when topically applied, it caused depigmentation of the epidermis [10].

HQ was shown to act as an inhibitor of tyrosinase in vitro, but in vivo it likely acts through the release of free radicals, which are toxic to melanocytes [11]. In 1981, Passi and Nazzaro-Porro showed that HQ acts as an alternative substrate for tyrosinase, whose oxidation product is the highly toxic metabolite 1,4-benzoquinone [12]. Other studies reported that the depigmenting activity of HQ results from its potent melanocytotoxic effects, which are mediated via its enzymatic oxidation to quinones [13–15]. Other enzymes, such as peroxidase, can metabolize hydroquinone resulting in toxic metabolites responsible for melanocytotoxicity [13, 16].

For many decades, hydroquinone has been recognized as the gold standard topical agent for skin lightening. Hydroquinone alone is of moderate to good efficacy for the treatment of most hyperpigmentary disorders. Epidermal melasma and post-inflammatory hyperpigmentation respond fairly well to topical hydroquinone, while dermal melasma and lentigines are not responsive. Efforts have been made to increase the efficacy of topical hydroquinone formulations by changing the vehicle as well as by adding other depigmenting agents. Alpha-hydroxy acids (AHAs), kojic acid, azelaic acid, etc., are examples of agents added to hydroquinone to enhance its depigmenting activity. A considerable increase in the depigmenting efficacy of hydroquinone was achieved by Kligman in 1975.

2.1.2 Kligman's formula

In 1975, Kligman and Willis investigated ways to enhance the depigmenting effect of hydroquinone [17]. It was found that the skin of acne patients treated with topical retinoic acid occasionally showed a light hypopigmentation after several months of use and that intradermal injection of corticosteroids into darker skin types resulted in depigmentation. These observations brought to the idea of combining HQ with retinoic acid and corticosteroids [17]. Surprisingly, this combination was found to have a synergistic depigmenting action. Retinoic acid promotes skin desquamation, therefore increases melanin loss from the superficial epidermal layers. In recent years, retinoic acid was found to be an inhibitor of glutathione S-transferase resulting in melanocytes becoming more susceptible to the cytotoxic effects of HQ [18].

Several studies demonstrated the superior efficacy of KF over HQ alone, resulting in KF quickly becoming the new gold standard. The KF has been modified over the years. Modifications of the initial formula involved changes in the types of corticosteroids and vehicles used. Modified Kligman's formulas (mKF) have become the most widely used HQ-based products for treatment of melasma [19, 20].

It is worth notice though that HQ nonresponsive pathologies, such as dermal melasma and lentigines, still remain unresponsive to the KF. The presence of retinoic acid in the KF counteracts to some extent the corticosteroid-induced skin atrophy. However, evident cases of skin atrophy after long-term use of KF have been reported [21]. In my hands, KF is an efficacious topical formula for the treatment of hyperpigmentary disorders, but at the expenses of a more irritant potential and of possible side effects with long-term use due to the presence of corticosteroids.

Most recently HQ became object of controversy as regulatory agencies around the world began questioning its safety. In Europe and in some Asian countries, hydroquinone has become unavailable due to concerns regarding carcinogenesis and melanocyte toxicity [22]. A study demonstrated that large amounts of oral hydroquinone caused cancer in rodents [23]. However, human being exposed to hydroquinone dust in hydroquinone factories showed a lower cancer rate compared with the normal population adding to the complexity of hydroquinone controversy. Adverse effects, such as skin irritation, contact dermatitis, and exogenous ochronosis, may occur with the unsupervised use of this compound. As a result of the controversy around the use of HQ, there exists a large and growing market for alternative products that are as effective in depigmenting the skin. Meanwhile, other formulations containing already existing depigmenting molecules, such as arbutin, kojic acid and azelaic acid, remained available, but unfortunately with a far less efficacy profile compared with hydroquinone formulations.

2.1.3 Arbutin

Arbutin is a HQ glycoside in which one molecule of D-glucose is bound to HQ. Its depigmenting effects result from the inhibition of tyrosinase. Many in vitro studies can be found in the literature showing arbutin's inhibitory effects on melanin synthesis [24–26]; however, the efficacy observed could hardly reach that of HQ. Several clinical studies have been performed in which arbutin was combined with other agents in formulations, e.g., niacinamide, bisabolol, retinyl aldehyde [27], or with tranexamic acid [28], showing to be as effective as 4% HQ in reducing pigmentation. According to some authors, arbutin is thought to work following its decomposition to HQ. Bang et al. report that arbutin can be hydrolyzed by the natural skin microbiota (*Staphylococcus epidermidis* and *Staphylococcus aureus*) leading to its conversion to HQ [29]. Others reported that arbutin can be converted into HQ by effect of UV radiation [30]. Thus, arbutin-containing skin lighteners are not totally HQ free. In addition, there are reports arguing that arbutin has pro-melanogenic effects in vitro, which obviously conflict with others reporting a depigmenting activity of arbutin [31]. Even if arbutin was as effective as 4% HQ, it is because it is actually converted to HQ. Therefore, there is no advantage in using arbutin instead of HQ.

On the other hand, as a dermatologist, arbutin-containing products in my hands are far less effective than HQ-containing formulations.

2.1.4 Kojic acid

Kojic acid (5-hydroxy-2-hydroxymethyl-4-pyrone) is a naturally occurring, hydrophilic fungal product obtained from various genera of fungi, such as the ones belonging to the genus Aspergillus and Penicillium [32]. It is a potent antioxidant, a tyrosinase inhibitor and a copper chelator, showing depigmenting effects in vitro [33]. A quick search on the literature confirms that at the moment there are no vehicle-controlled studies confirming the depigmenting action of kojic acid alone, in animal or in human trials. In an in vivo animal study on black Guinea pig skin, kojic acid did not show any depigmenting action when applied topically at 4% for 6 weeks (unpublished data).

When combined with other actives, kojic acid has been demonstrated to be effective in reducing hyperpigmentation, including melasma. A double-blind, split face study compared the efficacy of a gel containing 2% kojic acid in combination with 10% glycolic acid and 2% HQ to the same preparation without kojic acid for the treatment of epidermal melasma. Improvement of melasma was observed on both the facial sides, but higher efficacy was obtained with the gel containing the kojic acid [34]. Kojic acid is often combined with HQ for a synergistic depigmenting effect [32, 35]. Combination therapy including kojic acid may be an option in case a patient shows tolerability issues with other first-line therapies. However, kojic acid may be irritant and having sensitizing potential. Side effects reported following its topical application are contact dermatitis and erythema [36, 37].

2.1.5 Azelaic acid

In 1978, Dr. Nazzaro-Porro studied the mechanism of hypopigmenting effects in Pityriasis versicolor. At that time, a causative relation between the fungus *Pityrosporum* and hypopigmentation was suggested. It was postulated that certain metabolites secreted by the fungus might penetrate down the skin reaching the basal layer and damage melanocytes resulting in hypopigmentation [38, 39]. This hypothesis was confirmed, observations by electron microscopy revealed that melanocytes in the hypopigmented areas were highly damaged. Additional investigations followed showing that when *Pityrosporum* cultures were fed with unsaturated fatty acids with double bonds in 6–12 positions, dicarboxylic acids were produced. These metabolic products, including azelaic acid, were found to competitively inhibit tyrosinase in vitro [38]. Important observations suggest that medium chain-length dicarboxylic acids could be useful for treating hyperpigmentary disorders. Azelaic acid formulated in a cream was then used and showed good results in clinical studies on melasma patients first and later on patients affected by lentigo maligna [39, 40]. Histological analysis performed in the latter study shed light on the mechanism of action of azelaic acid, evidencing a progressive destruction of abnormal melanocytes followed by their replacement by normal ones. Further in vitro studies elucidated that azelaic acid has no depigmenting effect on normal melanocytes; instead, it has selective cytotoxic effect (inhibition of DNA synthesis and mitochondrial enzymes) in abnormal melanocytes [41].

Azelaic acid is a naturally occurring nine carbon C_8–C_{14} dicarboxylic acid produced by *Malassezia furfur* (formerly known as *Pityrosporum ovale*). Obtained from whole grain cereals, rye, wheat, and barley, azelaic acid has multiple functions; it scavenges reactive oxygen species, it has anti-inflammatory, antibacterial, comedolytic as well as anti-keratinizing properties, and last but not least, it inhibits tyrosinase as well as thioredoxin activities [39, 40, 42–44]. It is precisely because of these many properties that azelaic acid has been and is still used as a topical anti-acne agent [45]. Despite the fact that azelaic acid showed no depigmenting action in animal studies performed by Dr. Pathak et al. in 1985, [46] some human studies showed that very long treatment protocols (up to 24 weeks) could induce some depigmenting action in melasma lesions. In some of these studies, azelaic acid used for at least 6 months could show comparable effects to topical 4% HQ. The efficacy of a cream containing 20% azelaic acid has been compared with one containing 2% HQ in one study and with one containing 4% HQ in a second study involving 155 and 329 patients, respectively, both studies being 24-weeks long. Results showed that azelaic acid provides at least equivalent or, in the first study, even higher efficacy to HQ in the treatment of melasma [47, 48]. Side effects documented with topical use of azelaic include pruritus, mild erythema, and burning. Since azelaic acid is not cytotoxic to normal melanocytes, adverse events such as exogenous ochronosis or leukoderma are not associated with its use [48]. In addition, azelaic acid is not known to have mutagenic and carcinogenic potential.

In my experience, topical azelaic acid has a very long onset of action, which is not comparable with HQ or other effective depigmenting compounds, and this is associated with a very low compliance of patients who expect a depigmenting effect at least during the first weeks of application.

3. Newly emerging depigmenting agents

3.1 TXA in different forms

Tranexamic acid (TXA)—IUPAC name: trans-4-aminomethyl cyclohexane carboxylic acid—is a synthetic lysine analog well known for its anti-fibrinolytic activity. TXA has been used for several years to treat heavy bleedings, e.g., during menstruation or surgery as well as in case of trauma and bleeding disorders [49]. In recent years, TXA became more and more popular as a depigmenting agent. The first report describing the depigmenting effects of TXA dates back to 1979 [50]. The skin-whitening effects of oral TXA were accidentally found by Nijo Sadako, a Japanese investigator who had used TXA to treat patients with urticaria and observed improvements in their melasma. It has been postulated and later on reported that TXA is effective by modulating the vascular component of melasma [51, 52]. Recent studies have shown promising results on TXA for the treatment of melasma due to its ability to block melanin synthesis. Maeda investigated the mechanism of action of TXA in cultured human melanocytes. It was suggested that TXA inhibits melanin synthesis without interacting directly with melanocytes, but by interfering with the interaction between melanocytes and keratinocytes through the inhibition of plasminogen activator and therefore interfering with the plasminogen/plasmin pathway [53]. This results in a decrease of free arachidonic acid production and as a consequence melanogenic factors, such as prostaglandin and leukotrienes—which are known to stimulate tyrosinase activity—are reduced [54].

The paracrine melanogenic factor Endothelin-1 (ET-1) is generally increased in patients affected by melasma. In 2016, Kim at al. published about a possible mechanism of action of topical TXA in melasma patients. Topical application of 2% TXA resulted in ET-1 downregulation as shown in skin biopsies taken from the patients [55]. In addition, a slight decrease in the number of CD 31^+ blood vessels was also found in patients applying TXA. Additional literature aiming at elucidating the mechanism of action of TXA showed that it reduces tyrosinase protein expression as well as tyrosinase-related protein 1 and 2 (TRP1/2) levels [56].

TXA is a relatively new depigmenting agent, and it is used topically, by intradermal microinjection, and as oral agent for the treatment of melasma. TXA is an amino acid derivative, thus it does not adequately penetrate into the epidermis. A limited number of studies compared the efficacy of topical TXA at concentrations of 2% up to 5% to that of HQ (2–3%) alone or in combination with dexamethasone showing a comparable MASI score reduction with no statistical difference between groups [57–59]. The efficacy of the topical forms of tranexamic acid is rather controversial, and there is a need for large-scale, randomized controlled clinical trials comparing the efficacy of topical TXA versus oral or intradermal TXA [60]. However, the intradermal injection as well as the oral form of TXA tends to work as efficient depigmenting method for hyperpigmentary disorders.

A concern associated with the use of TXA for melasma has been the risk of developing arterial and venous thrombosis. The reported cases of thrombosis with oral TXA for the treatment of heavy bleeding refer to patients with risk factors for hypercoagulability, including clotting disorders, history of pulmonary emboli, prolonged immobility, hormone therapy, active bleeding, etc. [61–63]. This might be considered as a prohibiting factor for long-term use of TXA especially the oral form in patient with hyperpigmentary disorders.

To date, there are no studies comparing directly the efficacy of TXA with the one of triple combination cream (modified Kligman's formula).

In my hands, the topical form of TXA when not combined with other depigmenting molecules did not show any significant depigmenting results in patients with hyperpigmentary disorders. The intradermal form is quite effective, but is associated with pain, and most patients do not wish to continue the intradermal injections further than 4–6 months. The oral form of TXA is significantly effective in most patients with melasma, but is associated with a recurrence as soon as the treatment is stopped. Topical treatments proved to be ineffective in prohibiting such a recurrence.

3.2 Cysteamine

Cysteamine is the simplest aminothiol present in nature. It is an endogenous molecule resulting from the degradation of L-cysteine in mammalian cells during the Coenzyme A metabolic pathway [64]. Plasma concentrations of cysteamine are low, but it is highly concentrated in human milk. Cysteamine plays several key roles in human biology [65]. It acts as an intracellular antioxidant and has protective properties [65–67]. Cysteamine is orally administered to treat different pathologies, such as cystinosis and neurodegenerative disorders [67, 68].

The first evidence of the depigmenting activity of cysteamine dates back to 1966 when Chavin injected cysteamine hydrochloride into the skin of black gold fish model and observed a discoloration of the fish [69]. The higher depigmenting properties of cysteamine compared to HQ were demonstrated by two independent studies on animal models published by Frenk et al. and Bleehen et al., a couple of years later [70, 71]. Qiu et al. demonstrated that cysteamine exerts no cytotoxic effects on melanocytes and that it acts through melanogenesis inhibition [72]. Despite the high efficacy and high safety profile, two problems have precluded the use of cysteamine as a depigmenting agent: its instability and its offensive odor upon oxidation [65, 73]. These problems were overcome in 2012, and the first topical product containing cysteamine came to the market.

The first clinical evidences of the efficacy of topical stabilized cysteamine for the treatment of melasma were demonstrated in two double-blind, randomized, vehicle-controlled trials [74, 75]. The first trial involved 50 female melasma patients. At 2 and at 4 months, a statistically significant reduction in mMASI score (41.8% reduction at 2 months and 58.1% reduction at 4 months) as well as melanin index (47.2% at 2 months and 65.1% at 4 months) was observed in the group treated with stabilized cysteamine compared with placebo vehicle (mMASI: 7.1% reduction at 2 months and 10.8% reduction at 4 months; melanin index: 7.1% reduction at 2 months and 10.8% reduction at 4 months) [74]. The second vehicle-controlled study involved 40 melasma patients. mMASI scores were significantly reduced in the cysteamine group (55.6% reduction at 4 months) compared with placebo (7.6% reduction at 4 months). Melanin index measured by Mexameter and by Dermacatch was also reduced by 59.2% (versus 10% for placebo) and by 63.6% (versus 5.5% for placebo), respectively. Recent double-blind and randomized clinical trials compared the efficacy and tolerability of topical cysteamine with that of 4% HQ, TXA, and triple combination cream. When compared with Hydroquinone and TXA mesotherapy, stabilized cysteamine was shown to be as effective and better tolerated [76–79].

3.3 Mechanism of action

Cysteamine inhibits melanin production at different levels of the melanogenesis pathway by inhibiting tyrosinase and peroxidase, both essential enzymes leading to the conversion of tyrosine into dopaquinone and the further polymerization of indoles into melanin. Cysteamine is also a chelator of iron and copper ions, thus preventing Fenton-type reactions [80]. As an antioxidant and scavenger of free radicals, cysteamine suppresses all oxidation steps in the melanogenesis pathway also preventing photo-oxidation. Another interesting feature of cysteamine is that it is also able to increase levels of intracellular glutathione, amplifying natural depigmenting effects [81, 82]. In addition, cysteamine has the ability to cleave keratin disulfide bonds, thus enhancing the shedding of melanin in the corneal layer promoting epidermal turnover [76].

3.4 New formulations based on cysteamine

New formulations combining cysteamine with other molecules, such as certain vitamin B3 derivatives as well as with alpha hydroxy acids (AHAs) (cysteamine triple combination), recently entered the market. This triple combination was aimed at increasing the efficacy and accelerating the onset of action of cysteamine through the inhibition of melanosomal transfer by vitamin B3 derivatives and by increasing the epidermal penetration of cysteamine by AHA.

A very recent double-blind, randomized, and placebo-controlled 16-week long clinical trial has been performed to compare the efficacy, safety, and tolerability of the cysteamine triple combination with that of modified Kligman's formula for the treatment of melasma. Results are about to be published and showed an equivalent onset of action in terms of mMASI reduction and melasma/normal skin contrast reduction at 4 weeks post initiation of the treatment. Similar efficacy was shown at 16 weeks with no significant differences between the group applying the cysteamine triple combination and the group applying the modified Kligman's formula. No severe adverse events were reported in any groups.

Vitamin B3 group of chemicals in general confers anti-inflammatory, anti-pruritic, antimicrobial, and lightening effects. The latter results from the inhibition of melanosomal transfer. The combination of a vitamin B3 derivative with cysteamine exploits the complementary depigmenting action of the two molecules to achieve an additive depigmenting effectiveness.

An important advantage of cysteamine, in contrast to the gold standard triple combination (Kligman's formula), is the possibility of long-term use as a maintenance therapy. In addition, topical cysteamine is shown to be efficacious for the treatment of lentigines, which are usually resistant to most topical depigmenting agents [65].

It is possible that cysteamine triple combination could in the near future serve as a safe and effective long-term treatment for hyperpigmentary disorders in humans.

3.5 New oral and/or injectable treatments

3.5.1 Polypodium

Polypodium leucotomos (PL) is an anti-inflammatory, antioxidant, and photoprotective agent extracted from fern species [83–85]. These activities are attributed to the presence of several compounds in the extract, among others p-cumaric, ferulic, caffeic, and vanillic acids [86]. In 2004, it was shown that oral administration of PL (7.5 mg/kg) provided photoprotective effects in patients who were previously exposed to photochemotherapy [87]. The effect of oral PL extract (480 mg daily) was also assessed on pigmentation following visible light exposure in patients with Fitzpatrick skin type IV–VI for a period of 28 days. A significant decrease in persistent pigment darkening and delayed tanning were observed accompanied by a decrease in markers for cellular damage, suggesting that PL has depigmenting and cytoprotective effects [88, 89]. The clinical efficacy of PL was demonstrated also for the prevention and treatment of melasma. At 12 weeks, mean MASI score was significantly decreased in patients treated with PL as compared with placebo [90]. Another randomized and placebo-controlled clinical trial was performed with 40 Hispanic female patients with moderate to severe melasma, who were given either Polypodium (240 g doses, three times daily) or placebo for 12 weeks, both groups applied topical sunscreen (SPF 55). Both melanin index and MASI scores were reduced in both groups, and PL was found to have no significant depigmenting effect [91]. Another study was performed on 40 Asiatic patients with melasma comparing the combination of PL (twice daily, total daily dose of 480 mg) with topical 4% HQ and SPF50 sunscreen to the combination of HQ and sunscreen alone over a period of 12 weeks. Significant improvement in mMASI scores was observed for both groups, and at day 56, PL treatment was significantly better than placebo. The authors of this study suggested that PL is a useful adjunctive for treatment of melasma [92].

3.5.2 Grape seed extract

Grape seed extract (GSE) contains proanthocyanidin, a powerful antioxidant. Although there are no studies on the topical use of grape seed extract, oral intake for 6 months has been found beneficial in patients with melasma in a study conducted by Yamakoshi, et al. [93] L^* value and melanin index were measured. Both indices increased after 6 months of grape seed extract intake confirming the depigmenting action of GSE. The study suggested that GSE is effective in reducing hyperpigmentation in melasma patients. The depigmenting effects were only observed after 6 months with no further improvements afterward. The extract was shown to be safe and well tolerated. Another recent study on 30 women with mild-to-moderate facial melasma assessed the depigmenting efficacy of oral supplementation including GSE in combination with *Pinus pinaster*, vitamins, and minerals, used concomitantly with a high SPF sunscreen. MASI score decreased significantly at days 28, 56, and 84. A significant decrease in the melanin index between melasma affected skin and adjacent area was observed. Also a reduction in the number and areas of UV pigmented spots and in the areas of melasma was seen overtime [94].

Regarding the very slow onset of action, GSE might only be interesting as an adjuvant treatment for melasma in addition to topical agents and not as a monotherapy.

3.5.3 Glutathione

Glutathione (GSH) is a tripeptide of glutamate, cysteine, and glycine and is a powerful endogenous antioxidant. Endogenous GSH produces depigmentation by inhibiting tyrosinase and bypassing the production of eumelanin to that of pheomelanin [95]. At the time of authoring this chapter, only a few published clinical studies evaluated the efficacy of oral and topical glutathione as depigmenting agent. An open-label, 8-week study published in 2016 involved 30 healthy Filipino women, who were treated with a 500-mg buccal (sublingual lozenge) glutathione. The results showed a significant reduction in the melanin index (determined by Mexameter), and moderate lightening was observed in 90% of the subjects [96]. Topical oxidized glutathione (GSSG) at 2% was tested on 30 healthy women in a randomized, double-blind, split-face, and placebo-controlled study. Changes in melanin index values determined by Mexameter, moisture content of the stratum corneum determined by corneometry, smoothness, wrinkle formation, and elasticity of the skin were measured. The study lasted 10 weeks and showed a significant reduction of the melanin index in the GSSG-treated side [97]. The findings of these studies, however, need to be interpreted with caution due to some important limitations, such as the small samples size, the short study period, and no follow-up, no evidence of GSH efficacy on patients having hyperpigmentation but studies performed only on healthy subjects and lack of measurement of blood levels of glutathione. To date, there is no in vivo evidence on the efficacy of GSH on the treatment of hyperpigmentary disorders.

Systemic GSH through IV injection has been used as an off-label treatment for hyperpigmentary disorders and general skin whitening. This practice is forbidden by the FDA due to its hazardous side effects, such Stevens-Johnsons syndrome associated with IV injection of glutathione. The depigmenting action of IV GSH is not yet shown in any studies.

4. Conclusions

Topical cysteamine and tranexamic acid (intradermal and oral forms) are newer options that physicians can incorporate into their armamentarium. TXA, because of its demonstrated efficacy, is a good tool in hands of dermatologists for stubborn lesions.

The depigmenting efficacy of TXA and cysteamine has been evidenced in several clinical trials; however, additional larger studies are needed. To date, cysteamine has never been associated to severe adverse effects and thus represents an interesting alternative treatment to the Kligman's formula. If the results of the current studies showing the comparable efficacy of cysteamine with HQ and especially the Kligman's formula are confirmed in further clinical trials, cysteamine can be considered as one of the primary treatments for hyperpigmentary disorders. The absence of side effects associated with long-term use of cysteamine preparations suggests that it could be safely employed in the maintenance phase, since the Kligman's formula, although very effective for the acute treatment, is not a long-term option.

The existing risk of hazardous side effects such as thrombosis makes the long-term use of oral TXA risky. This causes TXA not to be considered as a long-term tool for the treatment of patients with recurring pigmentary disorders as melasma.

The other agents presented in this chapter, such as arbutin, kojic acid, and azelaic acid, are generally well tolerated, but appear having low efficacy and/or slow onset of action, although combinations of two or more depigmenting agents could improve that. More research and evidences are needed to demonstrate their individual benefits as well as optimal formulations.

Conflict of interest

Dr. Behrooz Kasraee is currently the president, shareholder, and the Chief Scientific Officer of Scientis SA.

Author details

Behrooz Kasraee
Swiss Vitiligo Center, Geneva, Switzerland

*Address all correspondence to: kasraeebehrooz2021@gmail.com

References

[1] Dabas G, Vinay K, Parsad D, Kumar A, Kumaran MS. Psychological disturbances in patients with pigmentary disorders: a cross-sectional study. Journal of the European Academy of Dermatology and Venereology. 2020;**34**(2):392-399. DOI: 10.1111/JDV.15987

[2] Witkowski JA, Parish LC. You've come a long way baby: a history of cosmetic lead toxicity. Clinics in Dermatology. 2001;**19**(4):367-370. DOI: 10.1016/S0738-081X(01)00196-1

[3] Lorenzi R. Mummy Shows Ancient Egyptians Bleached Their Skin—Seeker. 2016. Available from: https://www.seeker.com/mummy-head-shows-ancient-egyptians-bleached-their-skin-1851531742.html. [Accessed: May 31, 2022]

[4] Dyall-Smith DJ, Scurry JP. Mercury pigmentation and high mercury levels from the use of a cosmetic cream. Medical Journal of Australia. 1990;**153**(7):409-415. DOI: 10.5694/J.1326-5377.1990.TB125501.X

[5] Chan TYK. Inorganic mercury poisoning associated with skin-lightening cosmetic products. Cell. 2011;**49**(10):886-891. DOI: 10.3109/15563650.2011.626425

[6] CFR—Code of Federal Regulations Title 21. 2022. Available from: https://www.accessdata.fda.gov/scripts/cdrh/cfdocs/cfcfr/cfrsearch.cfm?fr=700.13. [Accessed: June 7, 2022]

[7] Oettel H. Naunyn-Schmiedebergs Archiv für experimentelle Pathologie und Pharmakologie. Die Hydrochinonvergiftung. 1936;**183**(2):319-362. DOI: 10.1007/BF01867498

[8] Martin GJ, Ansbacher S. Confirmatory evidence of the chromotrichial activity of p-aminobenzoic acid. Journal of Biological Chemistry. 1941;**138**:441-442

[9] Oliver EA, Schwartz L, Warren LH. Occupational leukoderma: Preliminary report. Journal of the American Medical Association. 1939;**113**(10):927-928. DOI: 10.1001/JAMA.1939.72800350003010A

[10] Peck SM, Sobotka H. Effect of monobenzyl hydroquinone on oxidase systems in vivo and in vitro. Journal of Investigative Dermatology. 1941;**4**(4):325-329. DOI: 10.1038/JID.1941.32

[11] Jimbow K, Obata H, Pathak MA, Thomas Fitzpatrick AB. Mechanism of depigmentation by hydroquinone. Journal of Investigative Dermatology. 1974;**62**:436-149. DOI: 10.1111/1523-1747.ep12701679

[12] Passi S, Nazzaro-Porro M. Molecular basis of substrate and inhibitory specificity of tyrosinase: phenolic compounds. British Journal of Dermatology. 1981;**104**(6):659-665. DOI: 10.1111/J.1365-2133.1981.TB00752.X

[13] Kasraee B. Peroxidase-Mediated Mechanisms Are Involved in the Melanocytotoxic and Melanogenesis-Inhibiting Effects of Chemical Agents. Dermatology. 2002;**205**(4):329-339. DOI: 10.1159/000066439

[14] Smith CJ, O'Hare KB, Allen JC. Selective Cytotoxicity of Hydroquinone for Melanocyte-Derived Cells is Mediated by Tyrosinase Activity but Independent of Melanin Content. Pigment Cell Research. 1988;**1**(6):386-389. DOI: 10.1111/J.1600-0749.1988.TB00140.X

[15] Ito Y, Jimbow K, Ito S. Depigmentation of black guinea pig skin by topical application of cysteaminylphenol, cysteinylphenol, and related compounds. The Journal of Investigative Dermatology. 1987;**88**(1):77-82. DOI: 10.1111/1523-1747.EP12465072

[16] Subrahmanyam V, Kolachana P, Smith MT. Metabolism of hydroquinone by human myeloperoxidase: Mechanisms of stimulation by other phenolic compounds. Archives of Biochemistry and Biophysics. 1991;**286**(1):76-84. DOI: 10.1016/0003-9861(91)90010-G

[17] Kligman AM, Willis I. A new formula for depigmenting human skin. Archives of Dermatology. 1975;**111**(1):40-48. DOI: 10.1001/ARCHDERM.1975.01630130042004

[18] Kasraee B, Handjani F, Aslani FS. Enhancement of the Depigmenting Effect of Hydroquinone and 4-Hydroxyanisole by All-Trans-Retinoic Acid (Tretinoin): The Impairment of Glutathione-Dependent Cytoprotection? Dermatology. 2003;**206**(4):289-291. DOI: 10.1159/000069938

[19] Sehgal VN, Verma P, Srivastava G, Aggarwal AK, Verma S. Melasma: Treatment strategy. Cell. 2011;**13**(6):265-279. DOI: 10.3109/14764172.2011.630088

[20] Rivas S, Pandya AG. Treatment of melasma with topical agents, peels and lasers: an evidence-based review. American Journal of Clinical Dermatology. 2013;**14**(5):359-376. DOI: 10.1007/S40257-013-0038-4

[21] Kasraee B, Mansouri P, Farshi S. Significant therapeutic response to cysteamine cream in a melasma patient resistant to Kligman's formula. Journal of Cosmetic Dermatology. 2019;**18**(1):293-295. DOI: 10.1111/JOCD.12837

[22] Draelos ZD. Skin lightening preparations and the hydroquinone controversy. Dermatologic Therapy. 2007;**20**(5):308-313. DOI: 10.1111/J.1529-8019.2007.00144.X

[23] Nordlund JJ, Grimes PE, Ortonne JP. The safety of hydroquinone. Journal of the European Academy of Dermatology and Venereology. 2006;**20**(7):781-787. DOI: 10.1111/J.1468-3083.2006.01670.X

[24] Boo YC. Arbutin as a skin depigmenting agent with antimelanogenic and antioxidant properties. Antioxidants. 2021;**10**(7):781. DOI: 10.3390/ANTIOX10071129

[25] Maeda K, Fukuda M. In vitro effectiveness of several whitening cosmetic components in human melanocytes. Journal of the Society of Cosmetic Chemists. 2006;**42**(6):361-368

[26] Maeda K, Fukuda M. Arbutin: mechanism of its depigmenting action in human melanocyte culture. | Journal of Pharmacology and Experimental Therapeutics. Journal of Pharmacology and Experimental Therapeutics. 1996;**276**(2):765-769

[27] Crocco E, Veasey J, Boin M, Lellis R, Alves R. A Novel Cream Formulation Containing Nicotinamide 4%, Arbutin 3%, Bisabolol 1%, and Retinaldehyde 0.05% for Treatment of Epidermal Melasma. Cutis. 2015;**96**(5):337-342

[28] Anwar AI, Wahab S, Widita W, Nurdin AR, Budhiani S, Seweng A. Randomized control trial outcomes of tranexamic acid combination serum as a depigmenting agent for the use in healthy individuals. Dermatologic Therapy. 2019;**32**(6):e13146

[29] Bang SH, Han SJ, Kim DH. Hydrolysis of arbutin to hydroquinone by human skin bacteria and its effect on antioxidant activity. Journal of Cosmetic Dermatology. 2008;**7**(3):189-193. DOI: 10.1111/J.1473-2165.2008.00387.X

[30] Chang NF et al. Study of hydroquinone mediated cytotoxicity and hypopigmentation effects from UVB-Irradiated Arbutin and DeoxyArbutin. International Journal of Molecular Sciences. 2017;**18**(5):969

[31] Nakajima M, Shinoda I, Fukuwatari Y, Hayasawa H. Arbutin Increases the Pigmentation of Cultured Human Melanocytes Through Mechanisms Other Than the Induction of Tyrosinase Activity. Pigment Cell Research. 1998;**11**(1):12-17. DOI: 10.1111/J.1600-0749.1998.TB00705.X

[32] Saeedi M, Eslamifar M, Khezri K. Kojic acid applications in cosmetic and pharmaceutical preparations. Biomedicine & Pharmacotherapy. 2019;**110**:582-593. DOI: 10.1016/J.BIOPHA.2018.12.006

[33] KAHN V. Effect of kojic acid on the oxidation of DL-DOPA, norepinephrine, and dopamine by mushroom tyrosinase. Pigment Cell Research. 1995;**8**(5):234-240. DOI: 10.1111/J.1600-0749.1995.TB00669.X

[34] Lim JTE. Treatment of melasma using kojic acid in a gel containing hydroquinone and glycolic acid. Dermatologic Surgery. 1999;**25**(4):282-284. DOI: 10.1046/J.1524-4725.1999.08236.X

[35] Deo KS, Dash KN, Sharma YK, Virmani NC, Oberai C. Kojic Acid vis-a-vis its Combinations with Hydroquinone and Betamethasone Valerate in Melasma: A Randomized, Single Blind, Comparative Study of Efficacy and Safety. Indian Journal of Dermatology. 2013;**58**(4):281

[36] Nakagawa M, Kawai K, Kawai K. Contact allergy to kojic acid in skin care products. Contact Dermatitis. 1995;**32**(1):9-13. DOI: 10.1111/J.1600-0536.1995.TB00832.X

[37] García-Gavín J, González-Vilas D, Fernández-Redondo V, Toribio J. Pigmented contact dermatitis due to kojic acid. A paradoxical side effect of a skin lightener. Contact Dermatitis. 2010;**62**(1):63-64. DOI: 10.1111/J.1600-0536.2009.01673.X

[38] Nazzaro Porro M, Passi S. Identification of tyrosinase inhibitors in cultures of Pityrosporum. The Journal of Investigative Dermatology. 1978;**71**(3):205-208. DOI: 10.1111/1523-1747.EP12547184

[39] Breathnach A, Levi-Montalcini R. The story of azelaic acid. A tribute to Marcella Nazzaro-Porro. Rendiconti Lincei. 1995;**6**(4):313-320. DOI: 10.1007/BF03001692

[40] Nazzaro-Porro M, Passi S, Balus L, Breathnach A, Martin B, Morpurgo G. Effect of dicarboxylic acids on lentigo maligna. Journal of Investigative Dermatology. 1979;**72**(6):296-305. DOI: 10.1111/1523-1747.EP12531744

[41] Nazzaro-Porro M. Azelaic acid. Journal of the American Academy of Dermatology. 1987;**17**(6):1033-1041. DOI: 10.1016/S0190-9622(87)70294-1

[42] Passi S, Picardo M, Zompetta C, de Luca C, Breathnach AS, Nazzaro-porro M. The oxyradical-scavenging activity of azelaic acid in biological systems. Cell. 2009;**15**(1):17-28. DOI: 10.3109/10715769109049121

[43] Sieber MA, Hegel JKE. Azelaic acid: Properties and mode of action. Skin Pharmacology and Physiology. 2014;**27**(Suppl. 1):9-17. DOI: 10.1159/000354888

[44] Schallreuter KU, Wood JM. Azelaic acid as a competitive inhibitor of thioredoxin reductase in human melanoma cells. Cancer Letters. 1987;**36**(3):297-305. DOI: 10.1016/0304-3835(87)90023-1

[45] Diane T. Versatility of azelaic acid (AzA) 15% gel in treatment of acne vulgaris: A review of clinical literature. Journal of American Academy Dermatology. 1016;**56**(2):AB18

[46] Pathak MA, Ciganek ER, Wick M, Sober AJ, Farinelli WA, Fitzpatrick TB. An evaluation of the effectiveness of azelaic acid as a depigmenting and chemotherapeutic agent. The Journal of Investigative Dermatology. 1985;**85**(3):222-228. DOI: 10.1111/1523-1747.EP12276684

[47] Verallo-Rowell VM, Verallo V, Graupe K, Lopez-Villafuerte L, Garcia-Lopez M. Double-blind comparison of azelaic acid and hydroquinone in the treatment of melasma. Acta Dermatology and Supplement (Stockh). 1989;**143**(143):58-61. DOI: 10.2340/000155551435861

[48] Baliña LM, Graupe K. The treatment of melasma. 20% azelaic acid versus 4% hydroquinone cream. International Journal of Dermatology. 1991;**30**(12):893-895. DOI: 10.1111/J.1365-4362.1991.TB04362.X

[49] Ockerman A et al. Tranexamic acid for the prevention and treatment of bleeding in surgery, trauma and bleeding disorders: a narrative review. Thrombosis Journal. 2021;**19**(1):1-16. DOI: 10.1186/S12959-021-00303-9

[50] Sadako N. Treatment of melasma with tranexamic acid. Clinical Report. 1979;**13**:3129-3131

[51] Na JI, Choi SY, Yang SH, Choi HR, Kang HY, Park KC. Effect of tranexamic acid on melasma: a clinical trial with histological evaluation. Journal of the European Academy of Dermatology and Venereology. 2013;**27**(8):1035-1039. DOI: 10.1111/J.1468-3083.2012.04464.X

[52] Masub N, Nguyen JK, Austin E, Jagdeo J. The vascular component of melasma: A systematic review of laboratory, diagnostic, and therapeutic evidence. Dermatologic Surgery. 2020;**46**(12):1642-1650. DOI: 10.1097/DSS.0000000000002770

[53] Maeda K, Tomita Y. Mechanism of the inhibitory effect of tranexamic acid on melanogenesis in cultured human melanocytes in the presence of keratinocyte-conditioned medium. Journal of Health Science. 2007;**53**(4):389-396. DOI: 10.1248/JHS.53.389

[54] Resende DISP, Ferreira MS, Lobo JMS, Sousa E, Almeida IF. Skin depigmenting agents in anti-aging cosmetics: A medicinal perspective on emerging ingredients. Applied Sciences. 2022;**12**:775

[55] Kim SJ, Park JY, Shibata T, Fujiwara R, Kang HY. Efficacy and possible mechanisms of topical tranexamic acid in melasma. Clinical and Experimental Dermatology. 2016;**41**(5):480-485. DOI: 10.1111/CED.12835

[56] Cho YH, Park JE, Lim DS, Lee JS. Tranexamic acid inhibits melanogenesis by activating the autophagy system in cultured melanoma cells. Journal of Dermatological Science.

2017;**88**(1):96-102. DOI: 10.1016/J.JDERMSCI.2017.05.019

[57] Ebrahimi B, Naeini FF. Topical tranexamic acid as a promising treatment for melasma. Journal of Research in Medical Sciences : The Official Journal of Isfahan University of Medical Sciences. 2014;**19**(8):753

[58] Banihashemi M, Zabolinejad N, Jaafari MR, Salehi M, Jabari A. Comparison of therapeutic effects of liposomal Tranexamic Acid and conventional Hydroquinone on melasma. Journal of Cosmetic Dermatology. 2015;**14**(3):174-177. DOI: 10.1111/JOCD.12152

[59] Atefi N, Dalvand B, Ghassemi M, Mehran G, Heydarian A. Therapeutic Effects of Topical Tranexamic Acid in Comparison with Hydroquinone in Treatment of Women with Melasma. Dermatology and Therapy. 2017;**7**(3):417-424. DOI: 10.1007/S13555-017-0195-0/FIGURES/10

[60] Bala HR, Lee S, Wong C, Pandya AG, Rodrigues M. Oral tranexamic acid for the treatment of melasma: A review. Dermatologic Surgery. 2018;**44**(6):814-825. DOI: 10.1097/DSS.0000000000001518

[61] Taparia M, Cordingley FT, Leahy MF. Pulmonary embolism associated with tranexamic acid in severe acquired haemophilia. European Journal of Haematology. 2002;**68**(5):307-309. DOI: 10.1034/J.1600-0609.2002.01607.X

[62] Krivokuca I, Lammers JWJ. Recurrent pulmonary embolism associated with a hemostatic drug: tranexamic acid. Cell. 2009;**17**(1):106-107. DOI: 10.1177/1076029609340902

[63] Calapai G. Systematic review of tranexamic acid adverse reactions. Journal of Pharmacovigilance. 2015;**3**(4):106

[64] Gallego-Villar L et al. Cysteamine revisited: repair of arginine to cysteine mutation. Journal of Inheritance Metabolism. 2017;**40**(4):555

[65] Desai S, Hartman C, Grimes P, Shah S. Topical stabilized cysteamine as a new treatment for hyperpigmentation disorders: Melasma, post-inflammatory hyperpigmentation, and lentigines. Journal of Drugs Dermatology. 2021;**20**(12):1276

[66] Hsu C, Ali Mahdi H, Pourahmadi M, Ahmadi S. Cysteamine cream as a new skin depigmenting product. Journal of the American Academy of Dermatology. 2013;**68**(4):AB189. DOI: 10.1016/J.JAAD.2012.12.781

[67] Besouw M, Masereeuw R, van den Heuvel L, Levtchenko E. Cysteamine: an old drug with new potential. Drug Discovery Today. 2013;**18**(15-16):785-792. DOI: 10.1016/J.DRUDIS.2013.02.003

[68] Thoene JG, Oshima RG, Crawhall JC, Olson DL, Sghneder JA. Cystinosis. Intracellular cystine depletion by aminothiols in vitro and in vivo. Journal of Clinical Investigation. 1976;**58**(1):180

[69] Chavin W, Schlesinger W. Some potent melanin depigmentary agents in the black goldfish. Naturwissenschaften. 1966;**53**(16):413-414. DOI: 10.1007/BF00625789

[70] Bleehen SS, Pathak MA, Hori Y, Fitzpatrick TB. Depigmentation of skin with 4-isopropylcatechol, mercaptoamines, and other compounds. Journal of Investigative Dermatology. 1968;**50**(2):103-117. DOI: 10.1038/jid.1968.13

[71] Frenk E, Pathak MA, Szabó G, Fitzpatrick TB. Selective action of mercaptoethylamines on melanocytes in mammalian skin: experimental depigmentation. Archives of Dermatology. 1968;**97**(4):465-477. DOI: 10.1001/ARCHDERM.1968.01610100105016

[72] Qiu L et al. Inhibition of melanin synthesis by cystamine in human melanoma cells. Journal of Investigative Dermatology. 2000;**114**(1):21-27. DOI: 10.1046/J.1523-1747.2000.00826.X

[73] Atallah C, Charcosset C, Greige-Gerges H. Challenges for cysteamine stabilization, quantification, and biological effects improvement. Journal of Pharmaceutical Analysis. 2020;**10**(6):499-516. DOI: 10.1016/J.JPHA.2020.03.007

[74] Mansouri P, Farshi S, Hashemi Z, Kasraee B. Evaluation of the efficacy of cysteamine 5% cream in the treatment of epidermal melasma: a randomized double-blind placebo-controlled trial. British Journal of Dermatology. 2015;**173**(1):209-217. DOI: 10.1111/BJD.13424

[75] Farshi S, Mansouri P, Kasraee B. Efficacy of cysteamine cream in the treatment of epidermal melasma, evaluating by Dermacatch as a new measurement method: a randomized double blind placebo controlled study. Cell. 2017;**29**(2):182-189. DOI: 10.1080/09546634.2017.1351608

[76] Desai S. Cysteamine: Clinical efficacy, safety and tolerability versus best-in-class treatments for melasma. The Journal of Cutaneous Medicine. 2021;**5**(6):s88

[77] Karrabi M, David J, Sahebkar M. Clinical evaluation of efficacy, safety and tolerability of cysteamine 5% cream in comparison with modified Kligman's formula in subjects with epidermal melasma: A randomized, double-blind clinical trial study. Skin Research and Technology. 2021;**27**(1):24-31. DOI: 10.1111/SRT.12901

[78] Karrabi M, Mansournia MA, Sharestanaki E, Abdollahnejad Y, Sahebkar M. Clinical evaluation of efficacy and tolerability of cysteamine 5% cream in comparison with tranexamic acid mesotherapy in subjects with melasma: a single-blind, randomized clinical trial study. Archives of Dermatological Research. 2020;**313**(7):539-547. DOI: 10.1007/S00403-020-02133-7

[79] Nguyen J et al. Evaluation of the efficacy of cysteamine cream compared to hydroquinone in the treatment of melasma: A randomised, double-blinded trial. Australasian Journal of Dermatology. 2021;**62**(1):e41-e46. DOI: 10.1111/AJD.13432

[80] Sakurai H, Yokoyama A, Tanaka H. Studies on the Sulfur-containing Chelating Agents. XXXI. Catalytic Effect of Copper (II) Ion to Formation of Mixed Disulfide. Chemical and Pharmaceutical Bulletin. 1971;**19**(7):1416-1423. DOI: 10.1248/CPB.19.1416

[81] Crinelli R, Zara C, Smietana M, Retini M, Magnani M, Fraternale A. BoostingGSHUsingtheCo-DrugApproach: I-152, a Conjugate of N-acetyl-cysteine and β-mercaptoethylamine. Nutrients. 2019;**11**(6):1416-1423

[82] de Matos DG, Furnus CC, Moses DF, Baldassarre H. Effect of cysteamine on glutathione level and developmental capacity of bovine oocyte matured in vitro. Molecular Reproduction and Development. 1995;**42**(4):432-436. DOI: 10.1002/MRD.1080420409

[83] Horvath A, Alvarado F, Szöcs J, de Alvarado ZN, Padilla G. Metabolic effects of calagualine, an antitumoral saponine of Polypodium leucotomos. Nature. 1967;**214**(5094):1256-1258. DOI: 10.1038/2141256A0

[84] Gomes AJ, Lunardi CN, Gonzalez S, Tedesco AC. The antioxidant action of Polypodium leucotomos extract and kojic acid: reactions with reactive oxygen species. Brazilian Journal of Medical and Biological Research = Revista brasileira de pesquisas medicas e biologicas. 2001;**34**(11):1487-1494. DOI: 10.1590/S0100-879X2001001100018

[85] González S, Pathak MA. Inhibition of ultraviolet-induced formation of reactive oxygen species, lipid peroxidation, erythema and skin photosensitization by Polypodium leucotomos. Photodermatology, Photoimmunology & Photomedicine. 1996;**12**(2):45-56. DOI: 10.1111/J.1600-0781.1996.TB00175.X

[86] Gombau L et al. Polypodium leucotomos extract: antioxidant activity and disposition. Toxicology In Vitro. 2006;**20**(4):464-471. DOI: 10.1016/J.TIV.2005.09.008

[87] Middelkamp-Hup MA et al. Oral Polypodium leucotomos extract decreases ultraviolet-induced damage of human skin. Journal of the American Academy of Dermatology. 2004;**51**(6):910-918. DOI: 10.1016/J.JAAD.2004.06.027

[88] Tasneem F. Oral polypodium leucotomos extract and its impact on visible light-induced pigmentation in human subjects. Journal of Drugs in Dermatology. 2019;**18**(12):1198-1203

[89] Nestor M, Bucay V, Callender V, Cohen JL, Sadick N, Waldorf H. Polypodium leucotomos as an adjunct treatment of pigmentary disorders. The Journal of Clinical and Aesthetic Dermatology. 2014;**7**(3):13

[90] Martin K, Caperton C, Woolery-Lloyd H, Avashia N. A randomized double-blind placebo controlled study evaluating the effectiveness and tolerability of oral Polypodium leucotomos in patients with melasma. Journal of American Academy of Dermatoloy. 2012;**66**(4):AB21

[91] Ahmed AM et al. A randomized, double-blinded, placebo-controlled trial of oral Polypodium leucotomos extract as an adjunct to sunscreen in the treatment of melasma. JAMA Dermatology. 2013;**149**(8):981-983. DOI: 10.1001/JAMADERMATOL.2013.4294

[92] Goh CL et al. Double-blind, Placebo-controlled Trial to Evaluate the Effectiveness of Polypodium Leucotomos Extract in the Treatment of Melasma in Asian Skin: A Pilot Study. The Journal of Clinical and Aesthetic Dermatology. 2022;**11**(3):14

[93] Yamakoshi J et al. Oral intake of proanthocyanidin-rich extract from grape seeds improves chloasma. Phytotherapy Research. 2004;**18**(11):895-899. DOI: 10.1002/PTR.1537

[94] Aladrén S, Garre A, Valderas-Martínez P, Piquero-Casals J, Granger C. Efficacy and safety of an oral nutritional (dietary) supplement containing pinus pinaster bark extract and grape seed extract in combination with a high SPF sunscreen in the treatment of mild-to-moderate melasma: A prospective clinical study. Cosmetics. 2019;**6**(1):895

[95] Villarama CD, Maibach HI. Glutathione as a depigmenting agent: an overview. International Journal of Cosmetic Science. 2005;**27**(3):147-153. DOI: 10.1111/J.1467-2494.2005.00235.X

[96] Handog EB, Datuin MSL, Singzon IA. An open-label, single-arm trial of the safety and efficacy of a novel preparation of glutathione as a skin-lightening agent in Filipino women. International Journal of Dermatology. 2016;**55**(2):153-157. DOI: 10.1111/IJD.12999

[97] Watanabe F, Hashizume E, Chan GP, Kamimura A. Skin-whitening and skin-condition-improving effects of topical oxidized glutathione: a double-blind and placebo-controlled clinical trial in healthy women. Clinical, Cosmetic and Investigational Dermatology. 2014;7:267-274. DOI: 10.2147/CCID.S68424

Chapter 6

Drug-Induced Pigmentation

Ivan Arni C. Preclaro

Abstract

Drug-induced pigmentation occurs in up to 20% of acquired pigmentary disorders of the skin. Association of its occurrence was reported in certain drugs, including alkylating/cytotoxic agents, analgesics, antiarrhythmics, anticoagulants, antiepileptics, antimalarials, antimicrobials, antiretrovirals, metals, prostaglandin analogs, and psychotropic agents, among others. Proposed mechanisms include (1) accumulation of melanin, (2) accumulation of drug, (3) generation of new pigment, and (4) deposition of iron. Though difficult to confirm the drug association, the history, with emphasis on currently used drugs, and clinical examination may guide practitioners to an accurate diagnosis. Treatment options include cessation of the drug, adequate sun protection, and non-ablative pigment lasers.

Keywords: drug reactions, pigmentation, drug-induced, pigment lasers, histopathology of pigmented disorders

1. Introduction

Pigmentary disorders are commonly seen in dermatologic practice that may have a negative impact on the quality of life of patients. In some of them, it may be brought by the use of certain medications leading to drug-induced pigmentation. The occurrence of drug-induced pigmentation has been estimated in 10–20% of acquired pigmentary disorders seen in the clinics [1]. Its incidence depends on the suspected medication, which varies from exceptional incidents to 25% of patients taking the medication [2]. Based on the literature, a number of reports have been attributed to be associated with developing drug-induced pigmentation. This includes alkylating/cytotoxic agents, analgesics, antiarrhythmics, anticoagulants, antiepileptics, antimalarials, antimicrobials, antiretrovirals, metals, prostaglandin analogs, and psychotropic agents, among others [1]. Despite the documented associations, the level of evidence supporting these has been variable. Most of these associations were reported in individual case reports and some case series. In addition, published systematic reviews have been limited; hence, the need for further prospective investigations regarding this disorder.

2. Pathomechanism of drug-induced pigmentation

The exact mechanism in the development of pigmentary disorders related to drug use is currently unknown. From the currently published papers, the evidence pointing to the pathomechanism of drug-induced pigmentation have been limited. Despite its occurrence in newer drugs, the deposition of pigments in the skin and mucosal surfaces has remained to be elucidated. With the advent of more sophisticated techniques, such as electron microscopy and mass spectrometry, further progress in its pathogenesis can be seen. Currently, there are four mechanisms proposed in the development of drug-induced pigmentation.

The first mechanism involves the accumulation of free melanin pigments in the dermis, or in the macrophages surrounding the blood vessels. This may be due to Ref. [1], the direct stimulation of the melanocytes by the culprit drug to produce melanin, [2] the inflammatory response to the culprit drug, or [3] the formation of a stable drug-melanin complex incapable of macrophage clearance [1]. Another mechanism implicates the accumulation of the culprit drug saturating the macrophages, which incapacitates its function to clear the foreign materials, or the culprit drug itself freely exists within the dermis as pigment granules [1]. Next, the culprit drug may influence directly the generation of new pigments, such as lipofuscin [1]. Lastly, the culprit drug may induce vascular damage within the dermis causing red blood cell extravasation and degradation, eventually leading to the deposition of iron [1].

These proposed mechanisms may not strictly explain the pathway in the development of pigmentation in each drug reported. With the development of new medications on the horizon, this may be accompanied by future perspectives on the pathogenesis of drug-induced pigmentation.

3. Clinical manifestations

The clinical picture varies for each drug based on the available reports. However, the sites of involvement, the pattern of pigmentation, and the color of pigmentation may help the clinician to suspect the culprit drug involved. The author divided the section into the pattern of pigmentation caused by drugs which is shown in **Table 1**.

3.1 Localized and diffuse pigmentation

There are many cases documented presenting with localized and diffuse pigmentation associated with medication use. Most of them usually start with a localized pigmentation evolving into a diffused pattern in the sun-exposed areas. The drugs more commonly described to cause pigmentary changes are clofazimine, amiodarone, minocycline, antimalarials, and chemotherapeutic drugs [3].

Clofazimine, an agent used in the treatment of leprosy, causes reddish-blue discoloration evolving into a violaceous to reddish-brown pigmentation. The pigmentation may be found in the skin and conjunctiva with prolonged use [5]. On dermoscopy, it shows yellow to white globules on a black background and honeycomb patterns [6]. Clofazimine-induced pigmentation resolves after months to years upon discontinuation [7].

Amiodarone-induced pigmentation has been well documented. It manifests with slate-gray to purple skin pigmentation found in sun-exposed areas, such as face, nose, and ears. The pigmentation appears after 6 months of administration and may be dose dependent. Patients who are taking more than 400–800 mg/day have a higher risk of developing pigmentation. It also may resolve upon drug cessation but in some cases, it persisted for up to 1 year [1, 8].

Distribution of pigmentation	Reported causative drug
Localized	Antimalarials, Tetracyclines, Amiodarone, Adriamycin, Tegafur, Antiretrovirals
Diffuse	Antimalarials, Tetracyclines, Amiodarone, 5-Fluorouracil, Cyclophosphamide, Adriamycin, Gefitinib, Sorafenib, Anticoagulants, Antipsychotics, Clofazimine, Antiretrovirals
Reticulated	Diltiazem, Paclitaxel
Flagellated	Bleomycin
Nail pigmentation	Antimalarials, Tetracyclines, Amiodarone, Clofazimine, 5-Fluorouracil, Cyclophosphamide, Adriamcin, Hydroxyurea, Sunitinib, Dapsone, Antiretrovirals
Mucosal pigmentation	Antimalarials, Tetracyclines, Antipsychotics, Amiodarone, Dapsone, Rifampin

Table 1.
Some drugs reported to cause pigmentation [4].

Minocycline, another established inducer of pigmentation, develops four characteristic clinical patterns. Type I shows blue-black pigmentation in the sites of previous inflammation or acne scars. Type II shows localized diffuse pigmentation in the anterior lower legs or in the photosensitive areas. Type III produces "muddy skin" presenting with diffuse bluish-brown to slate-gray pigmentation that can be aggravated by ultraviolet rays. Lastly, a noticeable pigmentation along the vermilion border of the lower lip. In addition, pigmentation of the other mucosal surfaces, such as conjunctiva, sclera, and nails, have also been described. Minocycline-induced pigmentation has a higher risk in the following: [1] those on prolonged treatment, [2] with a cumulative dose of more than 50 g, [3] with presence of other cutaneous inflammatory disorders, and [5] with co-administration of drugs that may induce pigmentation. Minocycline pigmentation occurs as early as 1 week of therapy up to 3 years after initiation [1, 8–11].

Chloroquine, hydroxychloroquine, mefloquine, and quinacrine are antimalarial drugs associated with drug-induced pigmentation. Its incidence occurs in one in every four patients taking these drugs. Generally, the discoloration is characterized by bluish-gray to deep purple shade of macules forming patches in the anterior legs and head that may progress into diffuse pigmentation accentuated in the photo distributed areas. In quinacrine-induced pigmentation, light yellow discoloration may be appreciated in the skin and mucosal areas. The pigmentation improves 2–6 months after drug cessation [1, 4, 12, 13].

Antipsychotic medications, such as phenothiazines (chlorpromazine) and tricyclic antidepressants (imipramine/desipramine), produce slate-gray to purple-gray pigmentation in the photodistributed areas, including the face and the extremities. Other affected areas include the nail beds and the eyes. The pigmentation happens over time and was associated with high cumulative doses. It was proposed that the antipsychotic medications, together with sun exposure, stimulate the melanocytes to produce melanin that results in discoloration. In chlorpromazine-induced pigmentation, the drug binds to the melanocyte to stimulate melanin synthesis. On the other hand, in imipramine-induced pigmentation, the drug or its metabolite may activate the enzyme tyrosinase subsequently increasing melanin production [1, 4, 14].

3.2 Reticulated pigmentation

Reticulated pigmentation has been described as "net-like" and "chicken wire" pigmentation with varying shades of pigments and unclear borders [15]. Drug-induced reticulated pigmentation was considered rare and was associated with some medications [16]. Diltiazem is a calcium channel blocker used to treat cardiovascular diseases. The development of diltiazem-induced pigmentation happens between 8 to 15 months from the administration of the drug. It was described as slate-gray reticulated pigmentation found in sun-exposed areas. Interestingly, the histopathologic findings reported were similar to lichen planus pigmentosus [17, 18]. Chemotherapeutic drugs, such as paclitaxel, cyclophosphamide, 5-fluorouracil, idarubicin, ifosfamide, and cytarabine, have also been implicated to cause reticulated pigmentation [19]. However, previous reports have used multiple chemotherapeutic drugs, and implicating its association in the development of reticulated pigmentation is quite limited [20].

3.3 Flagellate pigmentation

Bleomycin is a cytotoxic agent used to treat squamous cell carcinomas, testicular cancers, and lymphomas [21]. It is known to develop flagellate pigmentation that may be appreciated upon administration for up to 9 weeks. The pigmentation starts from erythema that can be found anywhere in the face, trunk, and extremities. It usually resolves after drug cessation and in some cases, it may persist up to 1 year later. In patients with more than 100 units of cumulative doses, the incidence of developing cutaneous reactions to bleomycin is around 8–20% [22]. Other medications reported with flagellate pigmentation include docetaxel, trastuzumab, peplomycin, and bendamustine [23–26].

3.4 Nail pigmentation

Drug-induced pigmentation of the nails may be due to the melanocyte activation in the nail matrix, or the deposition of the drug or its metabolites in the nail unit. Melanonychia usually results from the activation of melanocytes in the nail matrix. This produces streaks of longitudinal or transverse bands of brown to black stripes involving several nails [27]. Several medications have been reported to cause nail pigmentation which include zidovudine, 5-fluorouracil, methotrexate, cyclophosphamide, hydroxyurea, bleomycin, and daunorubicin. Melanonychia usually starts after 3–8 weeks of drug administration and resolves upon cessation of the drug between 6 weeks to months [28–30]. In some reports, the deposition of the drug happens in the nail plate. It may present with yellow tinted color of the nail plate in gold salts and tetracyclines while dark-brown to bluish-brown discoloration is associated with clofazimine and antimalarial administration [27, 31, 32].

3.5 Mucosal pigmentation

Mucosal pigmentation has been fairly documented in the conjunctiva and oral mucosa. This is more commonly documented in females and found in the gingiva, tongue, and buccal cavity. It presents with blue to poorly defined black pigmentation, which is promptly investigated to rule out the possibility of a mucosal melanoma [9, 33]. The development of drug-induced mucosal pigmentation may happen rapidly at onset or may take several days or years [34]. Its pathogenesis is still under investigation but may still be attributed to the proposed mechanisms mentioned [35]. Patients, who take antineoplastics, antimalarials, minocycline, and chemotherapeutic drugs, have a significantly higher risk of developing drug-induced mucosal pigmentation. Other drugs include zidovudine, golimumab, amlodipine, and clofazimine [36].

4. Diagnosis and assessment

The diagnosis of drug-induced pigmentation can directly be made on clinical grounds if the typical presentation of the pigmentation coincides with the exposure of the culprit drug especially with the known medications to cause drug-induced pigmentation. However, it may also be complicated due to insufficient evidence relating to the culprit drug, especially in the delayed onset of manifestations and the use of multiple drugs [37]. Given its complicated situation, the diagnosis for drug-induced pigmentation may be guided as follows:

1. A thorough patient history is recommended with emphasis on previous and current medications, including over-the-counter drugs and supplementation, and detailed medical history. If feasible, electronic medical records and previous pharmacy visits may aid the clinician in retrieving the drug list of the patient. It is important to take note of the common drugs that have been documented in the literature that may induce pigmentation. This includes antiarrhythmics, anticoagulants, antiepileptics, antimalarials, antimicrobials, antiretrovirals, metals, prostaglandin analogs, and psychotropic agents.

2. The onset and evolution of the lesions should be asked from the patient as keenly as possible. This should be done with a drug chart corresponding to the clinical course of the disease. It is important to note the changes in the intensity of pigmentation in correlation with the change in drugs as some drugs may be dose-dependent like amiodarone. An adverse drug reaction probability scale may help to assess the drug causality, such as the Naranjo algorithm [38].

3. Complete physical examination of the skin, nails, and mucosal surfaces is a must. The distribution pattern, morphology, and color may aid the clinician to suspect which drug may have caused the disease. Dermoscopic examination may be able to help distinguish other diseases that may present with odd pigmentation such as melanoma and hemosiderin deposition from a purpuric disorder.

4. Skin biopsy should be considered and may be correlated with the clinical picture. The location of the pigment, pattern of inflammation, and special stain patterns should be documented.

5. Differential diagnosis

Sun exposure has been the greatest contributory factor in developing pigmentary disorders and, coincidentally, a number of reports have documented the development of drug-induced pigmentation in sun-exposed areas. However, more common pigmentary disorders should have been considered first before thinking of

Melasma
Addison's disease
Hemochromatosis
Nutritional deficiencies (niacin and vitamin B12 deficiencies)
Ashy dermatosis or erythema dyschromia perstans
Pigmented contact dermatitis
Poikiloderma of civatte

Table 2.
Differential diagnosis of drug-induced pigmentation [1].

a possible drug-induced pigmentation in a patient. The list of differential diagnoses is included in **Table 2**.

Melasma is characterized by symmetrical hyperpigmented macules and patches on centrofacial and malar areas, especially in patients with skin of color. The factors contributing to its development include sun exposure, pregnancy, and hormone replacement therapy. Addison's disease presents with slate-gray pigmentation on both skin and mucosal surfaces. Pigmentation is accentuated in the flexural areas, scars, and areola. The diagnosis can be established with symptoms related to adrenal insufficiency and hormonal laboratory workup. Hemochromatosis should be considered in patients presenting with bluish-gray discoloration involving the skin and nails. This hereditary condition is usually accompanied by other diseases, such as diabetes mellitus, ophthalmologic problems, heart failure, and liver cirrhosis. Laboratory workups show abnormal levels of iron or copper and may be related to genetic mutations involving iron absorption.

Nutritional deficiencies, such as niacin and vitamin B12 deficiencies, may present with photodistributed pigmentation. Ashy dermatosis or erythema dyschromia perstans is a rare progressive disorder presenting with ash-brown discoloration predominantly seen in the trunk and proximal extremities. This condition may be hereditary and may be transmitted in an autosomal dominant way. Pigmented contact dermatitis is usually exacerbated by cosmetic products and is prevalent in middle-aged females of skin of color. It starts as erythematous pruritic patches progressing to diffuse and reticulated hyperpigmentation on face and neck. Poikiloderma of Civatte may also present with reticulated hyperpigmentation of the sides of the neck and V area of the chest. Factors contributing to the development of this condition include sun exposure, allergic reactions to fragrances/cosmetics, menopause, and genetic predilection [39]. Though histopathology may describe the deposition of some pigments in the skin, it is best to be correlated with the clinical information to arrive at the diagnosis of drug-induced pigmentation.

6. Histopathology of drug-induced pigmentation

Limited studies have correlated the histologic features with the clinical presentation of each drug class reported in the literature. This section will be discussing on the histologic findings of each drug class published. The histologic findings in each culprit drug-producing drug pigmentation mostly vary [40]. Generally, the epidermis may or may not show proliferation of melanin in the basal cell layer of the epidermis.

In the dermis, free pigment granules can be appreciated in perivascular and/or interstitial patterns. The pigment granules may show yellow-brown to black color. Some of these granules can be found inside the macrophages or adhere to the elastic fibers. The granules may have positive staining for Perls' method for iron, Masson-Fontana method for melanin, or both.

In minocycline-induced pigmentation, the histologic findings depend on its clinical variants. The type I and II variants show normal melanin pigmentation of the basal layer of the epidermis and the presence of golden brown to brown-black granules engulfed by macrophages in perivascular and periccrine patterns in the dermis. In type III variant, there is an increase in basal cell melanin pigmentation [41–43].

Amiodarone-induced pigmentation shows normal pigmentation of the epidermis with yellow-brown, lipofuscin-like granules surrounding the blood vessels in the dermis. These granules were positive for periodic acid–Schiff, Ziehl–Neelsen, Fontana, and Sudan black stains. At first, the granules were thought to be lipofuscin but recent findings support that the granules were amiodarone deposits in the dermis [44–47].

The histopathologic findings of pigmentation caused by the antimalarials, quinacrine, and hydroxychloroquine, show yellow-brown granular deposits within the macrophages scattered throughout the dermis and may be found extracellularly. However, the pigments in quinacrine-related pigmentation show a weak reaction or Perls' iron stain and negative for Masson-Fontana, while the pigments in hydroxychloroquine-related pigmentation show a positive reaction to Masson-Fontana and negative to Perls' iron stain [48, 49].

Antipsychotics, such as chlorpromazine, imipramine, and desipramine, demonstrate golden brown granules seen in the upper dermis surrounding the superficial vascular plexus. These granules are found within the macrophages. However, in imipramine and desipramine pigmentation, some granules are found floating in the dermis. The granules stain is positive for Masson-Fontana and negative for Perls' iron stain [50, 51].

In clofazimine-induced pigmentation, routine hematoxylin-eosin sections do not show any pigment deposits; however, birefringent red crystals can be appreciated in the fresh frozen sections. On fluorescence microscopy, these crystals are found surrounding large vessels in the dermis and show vivid red color. Interestingly, recent animal studies found that the crystals attributed to clofazimine pigmentation were from the separation of the free base form of clofazimine into the subcutaneous layer [52].

7. Treatment

Treatment strategies for drug-induced pigmentation have been limited. Avoidance and substitution of the culprit drug are the most reasonable option to treat drug-induced pigmentation. In some drugs, such as amiodarone, decreasing the dosage may help ameliorate the occurrence and severity of drug-induced pigmentation. In addition, sun protection, with the use of sunscreens, may avoid some drug-induced pigmentation brought by sun exposure from the use of certain drugs, such as antimalarials, antipsychotics, amiodarone, and tetracyclines [53]. Aside from sunscreens, physical barriers like umbrellas, hats, and wide-rimmed sunglasses should be advised, especially in patients at risk for intense sun exposure. Whitening topical medications, such as hydroquinone and hydroxy acids, have been found to be ineffective due to the location of pigment deposition in the dermis and/or adnexal structures [54].

Physical modalities, such as cryotherapy, have been documented in a case report of drug-induced pigmentation of the lip. A single cryotherapy session of open spray method using liquid nitrogen was applied for 30 seconds producing frost on the affected mucosal surface. Two weeks after, it produced a shallow ulceration which further improved 4 weeks after with minimal residual discoloration [55]. However, the improvement with the use of cryotherapy may be site-specific. The desired target in the dermis may outweigh the benefits of this modality, especially in the skin. Complications include scar formation, further pigmentary changes, and tissue disfigurement [56]. On a positive note, cryotherapy may be a good, cheaper alternative to lasers in drug-induced pigmentation of the mucosal surfaces.

Evidence supporting the use of lasers who may have failed or are unsatisfied with the current treatment option has been promising and may be an option for patients [54]. Conventional pigment lasers, such as quality-switched neodymium-doped yttrium aluminum garnet (Nd:YAG), alexandrite, and ruby lasers, have shown favorable results. Some studies have demonstrated good results in combining Q-switched pigment lasers with pulsed dye lasers or non-ablative 1550 nm fractional resurfacing lasers [57, 58]. These conventional pigment lasers induce photothermolysis of the pigment particles, making them less visible or promoting their clearance via recruitment and engulfment of pigments by phagocytic cells [59]. Frequency of treatment varies from a single treatment session of combination laser to multiple treatment sessions in single laser modality. This may suggest a combination of treatment strategies with the use of lasers may be more advantageous than single modality alone. Despite favorable reports of its efficacy, the optimal settings with the use of lasers have been variable. In addition, limited clinical trials have been published hence, the need for more studies such as prospective clinical trials.

Currently, picosecond lasers are cleared by the United States Food and Drug Administration in the treatment of pigmented disorders. It has been proven to be safer and more effective than nanosecond lasers in the treatment of dermal pigmentary disorders [60]. Several case reports and a case series have been published in terms of its efficacy in treating drug-induced pigmentation specifically to minocycline [61–64]. The frequency of treatment varies from a single session to five monthly sessions of picosecond lasers. All of them resulted in significant clinical improvement to complete clearance of pigmentation. Although the results were promising, further evidence is required to conclude its better efficacy than nanosecond lasers. Also, the lack of studies for other medications inducing drug pigmentation should reserve the use of picosecond lasers in the future and depend on the clinician's call.

8. Course and prognosis

Upon discontinuation of the culprit drug, pigmentation persists in most cases that may even last decades after drug cessation. This may result in an impact on the psychological and social aspects of each patient's life. Despite higher chances of persistence, drug-induced pigmentation is not associated with higher chances of mortality [65].

9. Conclusions

Drug-induced pigmentation is a rare, acquired pigmentary disorder brought on by various medications that have been used in our daily lives. Its development remains elusive but with the enhancements in research, the pathogenesis may be explained in the future. As clinicians, we have to keep in mind to include the possibility of drug-induced pigmentation in patients who have history of medication use. Prospective studies in the treatment of this condition may help clinicians to ease the burden on the patients' quality of life.

Acknowledgements

I would like to thank God and my family for the support they have given me ever since I took this field. I have my sincerest gratitude to my mentors, Professors Yu-Hung Wu, Wen-Hung Chung, Chun-Bing Chen, Chuang-Wei Wang, and the rest of the academicians and residents I have met during fellowship. You have inspired me to strive and grow in this field. Despite the struggles, I hope I can pass everything and grow with my younger colleagues in the Philippines just the way you have taught me. Lastly, our patients have been continuously reminding us that the field of medicine is a never-ending pursuit of excellence to deliver better care for them.

Conflict of interest

The author declares no conflict of interest.

Notes/thanks/other declarations

None.

Author details

Ivan Arni C. Preclaro[1,2]

1 Tondo Medical Center, Manila, Philippines

2 Dr. Jose N. Rodriguez Memorial Hospital and Sanitarium, Caloocan, Philippines

*Address all correspondence to: ivanpreclaro@gmail.com

References

[1] Dereure O. Drug-induced skin pigmentation. Epidemiology, diagnosis and treatment. American Journal of Clinical Dermatology. 2001;**2**(4):253-262

[2] Moore DE. Drug-induced cutaneous photosensitivity: Incidence, mechanism, prevention and management. Drug Safety. 2002;**25**(5):345-372

[3] Ghosh A, Das A, Sarkar R. Diffuse hyperpigmentation: A comprehensive approach. Pigment International. 2018;**5**(1):4-13

[4] Nahhas AF, Braunberger TL, Hamzavi IH. An update on drug-induced pigmentation. American Journal of Clinical Dermatology. 2019;**20**(1):75-96

[5] Karat AB, Jeevaratnam A, Karat S, Rao PS. Controlled clinical trial of clofazimine in untreated lepromatous leprosy. British Medical Journal. 1971;**4**(5786):514-516

[6] Chopra A, Mitra D, Agarwal R, Saraswat N, Talukdar K, Solanki A. Correlation of dermoscopic and histopathologic patterns in Leprosy - A pilot study. Indian Dermatology Online Journal. 2019;**10**(6):663-668

[7] Chavhan SD, Jawade S. Clofazimine induced pigmentation in leprosy patches. The Pan African Medical Journal. 2022;**42**:14

[8] Granstein RD, Sober AJ. Drug- and heavy metal--Induced hyperpigmentation. Journal of the American Academy of Dermatology. 1981;**5**(1):1-18

[9] Meyerson MA, Cohen PR, Hymes SR. Lingual hyperpigmentation associated with minocycline therapy. Oral Surgery, Oral Medicine, Oral Pathology, Oral Radiology, and Endodontics. 1995;**79**(2):180-184

[10] Tanzi EL, Hecker MS. Minocycline-induced hyperpigmentation of the tongue. Archives of Dermatology. 2000;**136**(3):427-428

[11] Katz J, Barak S, Shemer J, Langevitz P, Livneh A. Black tongue associated with minocycline therapy. Archives of Dermatology. 1995;**131**(5):620

[12] Skare T, Ribeiro CF, Souza FH, Haendchen L, Jordao JM. Antimalarial cutaneous side effects: A study in 209 users. Cutaneous and Ocular Toxicology. 2011;**30**(1):45-49

[13] Melikoglu MA, Melikoglu M, Gurbuz U, Budak BS, Kacar C. Hydroxychloroquine-induced hyperpigmentation: A case report. Journal of Clinical Pharmacy and Therapeutics. 2008;**33**(6):699-701

[14] Sicari MC, Lebwohl M, Baral J, Wexler P, Gordon RE, Phelps RG. Photoinduced dermal pigmentation in patients taking tricyclic antidepressants: Histology, electron microscopy, and energy dispersive spectroscopy. Journal of the American Academy of Dermatology. 1999;**40**(2 Pt 2):290-293

[15] Sinha S, Kulhari A. Reticulate pigmentary disorders: A review. Pigment International. 2019;**6**(2):67-76

[16] Masson Regnault M, Gadaud N, Boulinguez S, Tournier E, Lamant L, Gladieff L, et al. Chemotherapy-related reticulate hyperpigmentation: A case series and review of the literature. Dermatology. 2015;**231**(4):312-318

[17] Scherschun L, Lee MW, Lim HW. Diltiazem-associated photodistributed hyperpigmentation: A review of 4 cases. Archives of Dermatology. 2001;**137**(2):179-182

[18] Kubo Y, Fukumoto D, Ishigami T, Hida Y, Arase S. Diltiazem-associated photodistributed hyperpigmentation: Report of two Japanese cases and published work review. The Journal of Dermatology. 2010;**37**(9):807-811

[19] Kumar S, Bhattacharjee R, Kambhampati SBN, Narang T, Kanwar AJ, Vinay K. Chemotherapy-induced reticulate pigmentation in three Indian patients including a case in the pediatric age group. Indian Journal of Dermatology, Venereology and Leprology. 2021;**87**(3):386-388

[20] Cohen PR. Paclitaxel-associated reticulate hyperpigmentation: Report and review of chemotherapy-induced reticulate hyperpigmentation. World Journal of Clinical Cases. 2016;**4**(12):390-400

[21] Bennett JM, Reich SD. Bleomycin. Annals of Internal Medicine. 1979;**90**(6):945-948

[22] Lee HY, Lim KH, Ryu Y, Song SY. Bleomycin-induced flagellate erythema: A case report and review of the literature. Oncology Letters. 2014;**8**(2):933-935

[23] Cohen PR. Trastuzumab-associated flagellate erythema: Report in a woman with metastatic breast cancer and review of antineoplastic therapy-induced flagellate dermatoses. Dermatologic Therapy (Heidelb). 2015;**5**(4):253-264

[24] Mahmoud BH, Eide MJ. Bendamustine-induced "flagellate dermatitis". Dermatology Online Journal. 2012;**18**(11):12

[25] Tallon B, Lamb S. Flagellate erythema induced by docetaxel. Clinical and Experimental Dermatology. 2008;**33**(3):276-277

[26] Araki Y, Tamura K, Seita M. Side effects of peplomycin. Gan to Kagaku Ryoho. 1986;**13**(7):2446-2450

[27] Patel S, Tosti A. An overview of management of drug-induced hair and nail disorders. Clinical Practice. 2014;**11**:327-339

[28] Piraccini BM, Iorizzo M. Drug reactions affecting the nail unit: Diagnosis and management. Dermatologic Clinics. 2007;**25**(2): 215-221 vii

[29] Ledbetter LS, Hsu S. Melanonychia associated with PUVA therapy. Journal of the American Academy of Dermatology. 2003;**48**(Suppl. 2):S31-S32

[30] Oh ST, Lee DW, Lee JY, Cho BK. Hydroxyurea-induced melanonychia concomitant with a dermatomyositis-like eruption. Journal of the American Academy of Dermatology. 2003;**49**(2):339-341

[31] Hendricks AA. Yellow lunulae with fluorescence after tetracycline therapy. Archives of Dermatology. 1980;**116**(4):438-440

[32] Fam AG, Paton TW. Nail pigmentation after parenteral gold therapy for rheumatoid arthritis: "Gold nails". Arthritis and Rheumatism. 1984;**27**(1):119-120

[33] Ficarra G, Shillitoe EJ, Adler-Storthz K, Gaglioti D, Di Pietro M, Riccardi R, et al. Oral melanotic macules in patients infected with human immunodeficiency virus. Oral Surgery, Oral Medicine, and Oral Pathology. 1990;**70**(6):748-755

[34] Abdollahi M, Radfar M. A review of drug-induced oral reactions. The Journal of Contemporary Dental Practice. 2003;**4**(1):10-31

[35] Eisen D. Disorders of pigmentation in the oral cavity. Clinics in Dermatology. 2000;**18**(5):579-587

[36] Binmadi NO, Bawazir M, Alhindi N, Mawardi H, Mansour G, Alhamed S, et al. Medication-induced oral hyperpigmentation: A systematic review. Patient Preference and Adherence. 2020;**14**:1961-1968

[37] Gimenez Garcia RM, Carrasco MS. Drug-Induced hyperpigmentation: Review and case series. Journal of American Board of Family Medicine. 2019;**32**(4):628-638

[38] Naranjo CA, Busto U, Sellers EM, Sandor P, Ruiz I, Roberts EA, et al. A method for estimating the probability of adverse drug reactions. Clinical Pharmacology and Therapeutics. 1981;**30**(2):239-245

[39] Yoo J. Differential diagnosis and management of hyperpigmentation. Clinical and Experimental Dermatology. 2022;**47**(2):251-258

[40] Patterson J. Weedon's Skin Pathology. 5th ed. London, United Kingdom: Elsevier Health Sciences; 2020

[41] Simons JJ, Morales A. Minocycline and generalized cutaneous pigmentation. Journal of the American Academy of Dermatology. 1980;**3**(3):244-247

[42] Fenske NA, Millns JL. Cutaneous pigmentation due to minocycline hydrochloride. Journal of the American Academy of Dermatology. 1980;**3**(3):308-310

[43] Okada N, Sato S, Sasou T, Aoyama M, Nishida K, Yoshikawa K. Characterization of pigmented granules in minocycline-induced cutaneous pigmentation: Observations using fluorescence microscopy and high-performance liquid chromatography. The British Journal of Dermatology. 1993;**129**(4):403-407

[44] Trimble JW, Mendelson DS, Fetter BF, Ingram P, Gallagher JJ, Shelburne JD. Cutaneous pigmentation secondary to amiodarone therapy. Archives of Dermatology. 1983;**119**(11):914-918

[45] Haas N, Schadendorf D, Hermes B, Henz BM. Hypomelanosis due to block of melanosomal maturation in amiodarone-induced hyperpigmentation. Archives of Dermatology. 2001;**137**(4):513-514

[46] Miller RA, McDonald AT. Dermal lipofuscinosis associated with amiodarone therapy. Report of a case. Archives of Dermatology. 1984;**120**(5):646-649

[47] Ammoury A, Michaud S, Paul C, Prost-Squarcioni C, Alvarez F, Lamant L, et al. Photodistribution of blue-gray hyperpigmentation after amiodarone treatment: Molecular characterization of amiodarone in the skin. Archives of Dermatology. 2008;**144**(1):92-96

[48] Leigh IM, Kennedy CT, Ramsey JD, Henderson WJ. Mepacrine pigmentation in systemic lupus erythematosus. New data from an ultrastructural, biochemical and analytical electron microscopic investigation. The British Journal of Dermatology. 1979;**101**(2):147-153

[49] Puri PK, Lountzis NI, Tyler W, Ferringer T. Hydroxychloroquine-induced hyperpigmentation: The staining pattern. Journal of Cutaneous Pathology. 2008;**35**(12):1134-1137

[50] D'Agostino ML, Risser J, Robinson-Bostom L. Imipramine-induced

hyperpigmentation: A case report and review of the literature. Journal of Cutaneous Pathology. 2009;**36**(7):799-803

[51] Zelickson AS. Skin pigmentation and chlorpromazine. Journal of the American Medical Association. 1965;**194**(6):670-672

[52] Kossard S, Doherty E, McColl I, Ryman W. Autofluorescence of clofazimine in discoid lupus erythematosus. Journal of the American Academy of Dermatology. 1987;**17** (5 Pt 2):867-871

[53] Hassan S, Zhou X. Drug Induced Pigmentation. Treasure Island (FL): StatPearls; 2022

[54] Nikolaou V, Stratigos AJ, Katsambas AD. Established treatments of skin hypermelanoses. Journal of Cosmetic Dermatology. 2006;**5**(4):303-308

[55] Aktas H, Yilmaz OE, Ertugrul G. Cryotherapy for long-standing drug-induced lip pigmentation: A fast, safe and inexpensive procedure. Clinical and Experimental Dermatology. 2021;**46**(6):1130-1131

[56] Cook DK, Georgouras K. Complications of cutaneous cryotherapy. The Medical Journal of Australia. 1994;**161**(3):210-213

[57] Vangipuram RK, DeLozier WL, Geddes E, Friedman PM. Complete resolution of minocycline pigmentation following a single treatment with non-ablative 1550-nm fractional resurfacing in combination with the 755-nm Q-switched alexandrite laser. Lasers in Surgery and Medicine. 2016;**48**(3):234-237

[58] Riemenschneider K, Powers JG. Successful treatment of minocycline-induced pigmentation with combined use of Q-switched and pulsed dye lasers. Photodermatology, Photoimmunology & Photomedicine. 2017;**33**(2):117-119

[59] Bagheri S, Eisen D. Long-pulse neodymium-doped yttrium aluminum garnet laser treatment improves amiodarone-induced hyperpigmentation. Dermatologic Surgery. 2011;**37**(10):1539-1541

[60] Wu DC, Goldman MP, Wat H, Chan HHL. A systematic review of picosecond laser in dermatology: Evidence and recommendations. Lasers in Surgery and Medicine. 2021;**53**(1):9-49

[61] Sasaki K, Ohshiro T, Ohshiro T, Sakio R, Fukazawa E, Toriumi M, et al. Type 2 minocycline-induced hyperpigmentation successfully treated with the novel 755 nm picosecond alexandrite laser - A case report. Laser Therapy. 2017;**26**(2):137-144

[62] Rodrigues M, Bekhor P. Treatment of minocycline-induced cutaneous pigmentation with the picosecond alexandrite (755-nm) laser. Dermatologic Surgery. 2015;**41**(10):1179-1182

[63] Barrett T, de Zwaan S. Picosecond alexandrite laser is superior to Q-switched Nd:YAG laser in treatment of minocycline-induced hyperpigmentation: A case study and review of the literature. Journal of Cosmetic and Laser Therapy. 2018;**20**(7-8):387-390

[64] Moore M, Mishra V, Friedmann DP, Goldman MP. Minocycline-induced postsclerotherapy pigmentation successfully treated with a picosecond alexandrite laser. Dermatologic Surgery. 2016;**42**(1):133-134

[65] Writers AM. Examine the skin and thoroughly review medical/medication history when considering a diagnosis of drug-induced pigmentation. Drugs & Therapy Perspectives. 2019;**35**:418-423

Chapter 7

Skin Pigmentation and Cosmetic Considerations for Even Skin Tone

Anita Damodaran and Nirmala Nair

Abstract

The pigment polymer, melanin is the major determinant of visible pigmentation of skin, hair, and eyes. Its synthesis within organelles called melanosomes in melanocytes and transfer to and distribution within keratinocytes in the epidermis regulates skin pigmentation. Sunlight and its ultraviolet radiation component have a well-established role in skin tanning, through increasing epidermal melanin. Additionally, linked to the pigmentary system are disorders of pigmentation, resulting in problems ranging from hypopigmentation to hyperpigmentation. This chapter provides an overview of the prominent hyperpigmentary manifestations such as post-inflammatory hyperpigmentation (e.g., that associated with acne), solar lentigo, melasma, and peri-orbital hyperpigmentation and recent advances in cosmetic interventions borne out of strong scientific understanding and consumer clinical studies.

Keywords: hyperpigmentation, niacinamide, resorcinol, cosmetic, even skin tone

1. Introduction

Visual appearance is the reflection of one's inner self and is hence associated with self-esteem. To achieve skin devoid of imperfections has been an age-old quest, as it plays an important role in social acceptability. One such important aspect of appearance is skin color and its associated disorders. Skin color is determined by the amount and type of melanin (i.e., eumelanin and pheomelanin) synthesized in melanocytes and distributed within epidermal layers. It is also widely agreed that the type of melanin and its distribution in the epidermis are the most important factors in the protection of human skin from the detrimental effects of ultraviolet radiation (UVR). Constitutive skin color is what a person is born with and is genetically determined, while environmental factors such as UVR and pollution and physiological changes such as inflammation, hormonal changes, age, etc., influence facultative skin color.

Many constitutive pigmentation genes have been identified through spontaneous mutations causing a visible change in hair or skin color phenotype in mice or humans. All these genes are associated with either regulation of the pigmentation process in melanocytes or its development, survival, differentiation, and/or responses to stimuli [1]. In recent studies, using a genome-wide association approach complemented with targeted resequencing, scientists have identified previously unreported non-canonical skin pigmentation pathways in African populations, suggesting that the architecture of skin pigmentation can vary across humans subjected to different local evolutionary pressures [2–4]. Thus, novel variants in genes not previously linked to pigmentation are being discovered, and mounting evidence appears to suggest that there could be many more variants yet to be identified.

On the other hand, the molecular regulation of facultative pigmentation also called hyperpigmentation, has not been very well characterized. Limited knowledge exists on the etiology and the key genes/proteins involved in the induction, characteristics, and maintenance of the pathology of these conditions. Facial hyperpigmentary conditions like melasma, post-inflammatory hyperpigmentation (PIH), periorbital darkening, and solar lentigines (SL, age spots) are common cosmetic concerns across populations, especially in individuals of skin of color. Some of these conditions are described in the next section with the latest understanding of their underlying biology.

2. Hyper pigmentary conditions and biology

The common facial melanotic conditions prevalent in humans are shown in **Figure 1.**

2.1 Solar lentigines

Solar lentigines (SL) is a common hyperpigmentary disease occurring in approximately 90% of old Caucasians and 70% of old Asians [5]. It is reported to develop more frequently in men than women [6, 7]. It presents a well-demarcated circumscribed yellow or brown macule with a diameter of 1–3 cm, predominantly on sun-exposed areas such as the face and the dorsal aspects of the hands and forearms [8]. However, unlike UV tanning, which may disappear with time in the absence of further sun exposure, SL is not known to resolve on its own, probably due to irreversible damage resulting from repeated sun exposure. Besides sun exposure, environmental factors such as constituents of ambient air pollution; may also contribute to SL development [9].

Histopathological assessment of SL has been carried out by several independent investigators. Prominent features include hyperpigmentation of the basal cell layer with a characteristic club-shaped elongation of rete ridges, numerous melanocytes, and increased melanin production without cellular atypia. A significant increase in both the epidermal area and the number of melanocytes, compared to that with a similar degree of photodamage, but frequently lacking the rete ridge hyperplasia classically

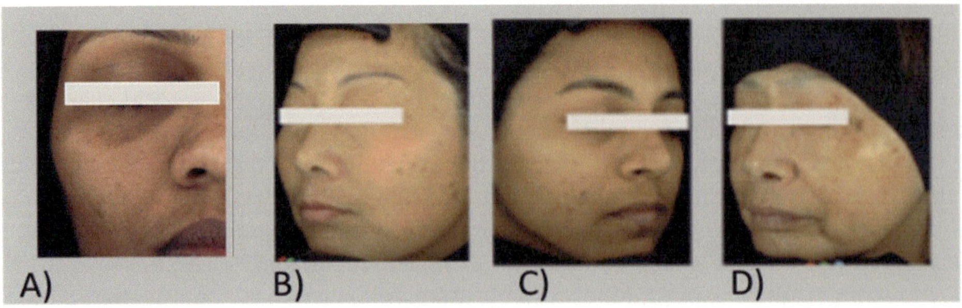

Figure 1.
Various facial hyper melanosis prevalent in humans. (A) Periorbital hyperpigmentation (POH); (B) solar/senile lentigines (SL); (C) post inflammatory hyperpigmentation (PIH); (D) melasma.

associated with lentigines from other anatomic sites have been reported for facial SL [10, 11]. Classification of human SL progressive stages, based on the degree of melanin deposition and the depth and complexity of the rete ridges has been proposed with early stages of SL presenting with lower melanin levels as well as shorter and simpler rete ridges, whereas later stages show an accumulation of melanin and intricated rete ridges protruding into the thinning dermis and epidermis [12–14]. More recent studies have also pointed to the role of underlying inflammation in SL pathogenesis [15].

In recent years, insights generated through several qualitative and quantitative studies have significantly advanced our understanding of the underlying mechanisms in SL pathogenesis. Gene profiling studies reported upregulation of genes related to inflammation, fatty-acid metabolism, and melanogenesis, and downregulation of cornified envelope-related genes, indicating that solar lentigo is likely induced by mutagenic effects of repeated ultraviolet light exposures, thereby increasing melanin production, with a concomitant reduction in proliferation and differentiation of keratinocytes [14, 16]. The observed reduction in keratinocyte proliferation has been corroborated in a subsequent study, wherein the authors propose that early events may involve pigment-related genes, but with increasing time, increased levels of keratins 5 and 10 may put pressure on the basement membrane with basal keratinocytes loaded with melanin, pushing down toward the dermis to form rete ridges instead of moving upwards toward the stratum corneum as in normal skin [17]. Analysis of 160 skin biopsy samples from the lesional skin of SL showed a gradual increase in the expression of specific microRNAs from photo protected to peri-lesional skin to SL [18]. The profile reveals a significant change in microRNAs that regulate genes involved in lipid and fatty acid metabolism as well as inflammation.

Several independent studies have implicated cell types besides melanocytes in SL pathogenesis. In a study to decipher morphological and immunohistochemical changes of keratinocytes in facial SL, it was shown that individual keratinocytes were larger in size and showed increased p16 staining, pointing to a role for senescent changes underlying the pathogenesis [19]. More recently, in a study on 190 SL subjects, *Notch1*-dependent keratinocyte malfunction was suggested as the cause of the development of SL [20]. Besides the epidermal compartment, several independent studies have also reported changes in epithelial-mesenchymal crosstalk in SL pathogenesis. Prominent among these are endothelin-1 (*ET-1*), hepatocyte growth factor (*HGF*), keratinocyte growth factor (*KGF*), and stem cell factor (*SCF*) [21, 22]. An interesting difference between UVB melanosis and SL is that in the former, *ET-1* and *SCF* are stimulated by interleukin-1 alpha (*IL-1α*), while in SL, they are stimulated by tumor necrosis factor-alpha (*TNFα*) [23]. Observed degradation of heparan sulfate chains owing to increased heparinase at the dermal-epidermal junction (DEJ), may exacerbate the transfer of growth factors and cytokines between the epidermis and dermis, contributing to hyperpigmentation in SL [24]. Studies have also pointed to increased blood flow and vasculature in SL using immunohistochemistry [25], 3D microvascular analysis [26], and optical coherence tomography angiography [27]. Most recently, a dysregulation of *Nrf2* signaling has been shown to be associated with SL pathogenesis [28]. Taken together, these pieces of evidence point to a complex network of cells and secreted factors that are likely involved in the development and progression of SL.

2.2 Postinflammatory hyperpigmentation

Postinflammatory hyperpigmentation (PIH) is one of the most common causes of altered normal skin color [29]. It is an acquired hyper-melanosis and a common sequela of various inflammatory episodes. It primarily afflicts patients with darker skin types (Fitzpatrick types III–VI), although all skin types can develop PIH [30]. As compared to 25% in white patients, the prevalence of PIH in Hispanic and black patients is 48 and 65%, respectively [31]. Additionally, it has been reported to occur with equal incidence in males and females of all ages [32]. Although PIH is easily diagnosed from the patient's history and the presence of inflammation, several dermatoses lead to PIH without noticeable inflammation. Hence, while visual assessment can aid in PIH evaluation, the use of non-invasive methods can further aid diagnosis [33].

PIH presents itself in two forms—epidermal (light to dark brown) which usually disappears spontaneously and dermal (blue-gray coloration) which has a more prolonged course and may either take years to resolve or may be permanent [33, 34]. Unfortunately, a vicious cycle may emerge leading to new areas of hyperpigmentation if the underlying inflammatory disorder is not resolved [34]. In many cases, the extent of damage to the skin may result in scars and keloids.

Causative factors can be divided into endogenous and exogenous factors. The former includes PIH from inherited diseases such as incontinentia pigmenti, cutaneous diseases such as acne, lichen planus, erythema dyschromia persistans, and facial melanoses, as well as systemic diseases such as morphea, porphyria, and biliary cirrhosis [29]. The latter on the other hand include mechanical trauma, extremes of temperature, ionizing and non-ionizing radiation, phototoxic reactions, laser resurfacing [35, 36], and cases of contact dermatitis [37]. Noteworthy is the PIH commonly accompanying acne, often considered more bothersome than acne itself [38] and that accompanying axillary darkening because of shaving, plucking, and/or antiperspirant use [39].

Different histological patterns of PIH emerge, depending on which skin layer is involved. For the epidermal type, there appears to be an increase in the number (hyperplasia), size (hypertrophy), and activity of melanocytes, leading to increased melanin content, with little dermal changes [40]. On the other hand, in the dermal type, melanin enters the dermis, contributing to dermal pigmentation, with an accompanying perivascular lymphocytic infiltrate [40, 41].

Likely pathogenic mechanisms underlying PIH include inflammatory mediators such as arachidonic acid metabolites, nitric oxide, etc., and crosstalk between melanocytes and neighboring keratinocytes and fibroblasts, resulting in the exchange of several melanogenic factors [42].

2.3 Periorbital hyperpigmentation

Periorbital hyperpigmentation (POH) is a common dermatological condition that presents as a dark periorbital area beneath or around the eyes. While it afflicts about 78% of the global population, the majority of the affected individuals are of Asian and African origin [43]. It is reported to occur in both sexes with a greater frequency in females with early onset at age 16–25 [44, 45]. It can also frequently be seen in multiple members of the same family [46].

While the etiology is multifactorial, prominent causative factors include familial, UV, inadequate sleep, post-inflammatory hyperpigmentation following atopic dermatitis, allergic contact dermatitis, lichen planus pigmentosus, erythema dyschromicum perstans [47] tear-trough depression, and periorbital edema [43, 48, 49]. Basis the clinical pattern of pigmentation and vasculature, POH can be classified into (a) constitutional, which involves the presence of a curved band of dark brown to black pigmentation on the skin of the lower eyelids, (b) postinflammatory pigmentation, marked by the presence of irregular patches of dark brownish or gray pigmentation on the skin of the lower, upper, or both the eyelids with lichenifed eczema in surrounding areas, (c) vascular, involving bluish discoloration of the lower eyelids and visible greenish blue veins that become more prominent on stretching of the overlying skin, (d) the shadow effect, involving the presence of deep tear trough over the medial aspect of the inferior orbital rim that disappears with direct lighting, and (e) mixed highlighted by presence of periorbital blue, purple, or pink hue with puffiness associated with palpebral bags, blepharoptosis, and loss of fat with bony prominence [43, 50, 51].

The pathogenesis of POH may be due to one of many factors, notably, dermal melanocytosis [52], an extension of pigmentary demarcation lines of the face [45], postinflammatory hyperpigmentation, superficial location of the vasculature [53], tear-trough depression [52], and thinning of skin [54]. Ultraviolet-induced damage stimulates melanogenesis through multiple pathways [55] or melasma, if it appears on the eyelids, leading to dark eyelids and a tanned lower eyelid region [56].

Histological examination reveals that the most consistent features of POH are hyper melanization of the basal layer and lower malpighian layer with increased melanin granules together with dermal melanin incontinence, dermal melanophages, and perivascular lymphocytic infiltrate [53, 57, 58]. Additionally, the dilation of dermal blood vessels may contribute to the severity of POH [58]. In a study on Asian subjects, the group reported dermal melanocytosis along with melanophages in patients with POH as detected by immune-histochemical staining with S-100 antigen [59]. The almost universal presence of dermal melanin is likely to influence poor treatment outcomes of POH.

Recently, in a study on Caucasian, Asian, and African subjects, it was confirmed through various instrumental measurements that the three features associated with the occurrence of infraorbital dark circles, were hyperpigmentation, a tendency for more dilated, thicker, or increased number of capillaries and thinner skin in the under-eye area in Caucasian subjects. These trends were also observed in the African and far east Asian subjects [60]. However, detailed molecular mechanisms involved in POH continue to elude us.

2.4 Melasma

Melasma is defined as a chronic, acquired disorder of hyperpigmentation, presenting as symmetrical, light to dark brown and ashen gray-brown macules and patches on sun-exposed areas of the face and neck [61]. It is also sometimes referred to in medical literature as the "mask of pregnancy or chloasma," the latter originating from the Greek word chloazein, meaning to be green [62]. It is primarily a disease of adult women, with reported cases in men being only 10% [63], presenting mostly in the facial area of darker-complexioned individuals (skin types IV–VI) of Hispanic, East Asian, and Southeast Asian origin exposed to intense ultraviolet radiation [62] and shorter wavelengths of visible light [64]. In a multicenter survey from nine countries, the mean onset of age was 34 years [65]. It negatively impacts the quality of life; often, poor therapeutic responses pose a huge challenge to dermatologists and escalate the cost of treatment for affected individuals [66]. Predisposing factors include pregnancy, hormonal therapies (including oral contraceptives), phototoxic and anti-epileptic medications, intense sun exposure [67], and genetic predisposition [68, 69]. Recent studies suggest that thyroid hormones may play a key role in melasma [70].

There are two broad ways to classify melasma: (a) based on the distribution of lesions, three clinical patterns of melasma have been recognized—Centro facial, malar, and mandibular; (b) based on the distribution of melanin in the epidermis and dermis using a Woods lamp into epidermal, dermal, mixed, and indeterminate types [62].

As with other hyperpigmentary conditions, the pathogenesis is multifactorial and poorly understood. Some of the prominently reported mechanisms underlying melasma pathogenesis include melanocyte activation, melanin and melanosome retention in the epidermis and dermis, basement membrane damage, solar elastosis, increased mast cell count and increased vascularization [71]. Overall, the epidemiological and pathophysiological data seem to suggest that melasma is a photoaging disorder [64].

Transcriptional profiling revealed that a subset of *Wnt* signaling modulators, including *Wnt* inhibitory factor-1 (*WIF-1*), secreted frizzled-related protein 2 (*sFRP2*), and *Wnt5a*, were upregulated in lesional melasma skin [72]. The down-regulation of *WIF-1* which may occur in keratinocytes and fibroblasts can influence melasma pathogenesis through the up-regulation of canonical and non-canonical *Wnt* signaling [73]. Given that UV is implicated in melasma pathogenesis, the upregulation of several of the UV-induced cytokines in melasma is not surprising.

Likewise, melanocytes in melasma can also be activated by hormones. Notably, lesional skin shows increased expression of progesterone receptors [74, 75] and estrogen receptor beta expression in the dermis [74]. Significant advances have been made in elucidating the influence of estrogens on melanogenesis [76].

The number of blood vessels, vessel size, and vessel density are greater in lesional melasma skin than in perilesional skin [77–79]. Factors that could influence vascularization and pigmentation in melasma are upregulated in lesional areas of melasma. Prominent among these are vascular endothelial growth factor (*VEGF*), stem cell factor (*SCF*), and inducible nitric oxide synthase (*iNOs*) [77, 80, 81]. Endothelin-1 (*ET-1*) released from endothelial cells stimulates pigmentation through endothelin receptor B activation at the surface of melanocytes [82]. Concerning solar elastosis, the current consensus is that 83–93% of melasma patients show a variable degree of solar elastosis with abnormal elastotic material [83, 84]. An increased number of mast cells, particularly around elastotic areas of the dermis in lesional melasma [83] is believed to exacerbate solar elastosis, besides promoting basement membrane disruption and extracellular matrix (ECM) degradation through the release of tryptase, vascular endothelial growth factor (*VEGF*), fibroblast growth factor (*FGF*)-2, and transforming growth factor-beta (*TGF-β*) [85].

Basement membrane damage has been reported in melasma patients via periodic acid-Schiff-diastase (D-PAS) staining and anti-collagen type IV immunohistochemistry, respectively [84]. This predisposes melanocytes to hang into the dermal compartment—the characteristic pendulous melanocytes observed in histology leading to dermal incontinence [86]. Increased expression of matrix metalloproteinases such as *MMP2* and *9* in response to chronic UV exposure is likely to contribute to basement membrane damage [87]. The outcomes of these events result in melanin or melanophages in the dermis [84, 88]. Recently, melanin content, location and distribution in melasma, and elastosis severity were confirmed using multiphoton microscopy [89]. Dermal incontinence is a challenge across hyperpigmentation and one, that is likely to significantly contribute to the recalcitrant nature of these conditions.

While we continue to investigate the pathology and biology of various hyperpigmentary conditions, the other key question that needs to be addressed is the factors that make an individual susceptible to a particular hyperpigmentary disorder, besides family history. An in-depth analysis of the epidemiology and population genetics data may help in identifying key population or individual biology, which will in turn support the designing of better preventive options.

3. Role of UV and visible light in skin pigmentation

From the discussion on hyperpigmentary disorders prevalent in humans in the previous section, the role of UV is quite evident and seems to be central to all conditions, so it is worthwhile to discuss the effects of UV and solar spectrum on the skin in the following section.

Ultraviolet radiation on the earth's surface, both UVB and UVA radiation, constitutes about 5% of total sunlight received. In skin phototypes I–II, exposure to UVB radiation, leads to erythema and sunburns [90]. Skin pigmentation or tanning induced by UV radiation in skin phototypes III–IV, occurs in three different phases-immediate pigment darkening (IPD) and persistent pigment darkening (PPD), both thought to be the result of oxidation or redistribution of melanin while delayed tanning (DT), a characteristic of UVB is because of new melanin synthesis [91, 92]. There is limited data on the skin types V–VI and their response behavior to UV. While erythema, IPD, and DT are the noticeable effects of UV-induced damage to the skin in a short period, repeated exposure may result in one of the chronic effects of sun exposure such as photo-aging which results in the development of deep wrinkles and spots on the exposed skin [93].

UVB (290–320 nm) being more energetic directly damages DNA by causing cyclobutane pyrimidine dimerization and the formation of 6–4 photoproducts. UVA rays (320–400 nm) on the other hand generate reactive oxygen species (ROS) that, in turn, cause indirect DNA damage and activation of several cellular pathways [94]. At the molecular level, UV has been shown to cause DNA damage with subsequent accumulation of *p53* protein which regulates the expression of the transcription factor hepatocyte nuclear factor-1α in melanocytes, which in turn regulates *MITF* and tyrosinase levels [95] and the transcription of the pro-opiomelanocortin (*POMC*) gene in keratinocytes which eventually regulates *MC1R* induced melanogenesis in melanocytes [96]. GWAS, linkage, and association-based studies on European and non-European populations suggest the role of distinct genes like glutamate metabotropic receptor 6 (*GRM6*), activating transcription factor 1 *(ATF1)*, *WNT1*, and pre melanosome protein 17 *(SILV/Pmel17)* in observed differential tanning response [1, 97] pointing to the fact that the genetic makeup of the population could drive the nature and the molecular events leading to a tan.

In the past decade, the focus has shifted to the other wavelengths of light namely visible light (400–700 nm) and infrared radiation (IR; 700–1400 nm) which form a major part of the solar spectrum, 45 and 54%, respectively. These longer wavelengths penetrate deeper into the skin and can induce ROS and potentially cause erythema in light skin and pigmentary changes in individuals with darker skin types [92, 98–101]. Furthermore, susceptibility to pigmentation by visible and IR radiation was shown to reside in darker skin types more than Caucasian skin [92, 102, 103]. Visible light and IR activate metalloproteinases and decrease collagen production by inducing oxidative stress [104, 105]. Damodaran et al. [106] demonstrated that among variable parts of the visible light spectrum, blue wavelength contributes maximally to pigmentation in human subjects (**Figure 2A** and **B**). As the blue region is adjacent to UV radiation in terms of wavelength and frequency, blue light is expected to induce photobiological effects like UV radiation, including photoaging and skin pigmentation [101, 107]. In the field of ophthalmology, researchers have identified that "excessive blue light exposure" may cause photokeratitis and retinal injury [108]. Interestingly, the prevalence of photoreceptors like opsins, which recognize blue and green wavelengths of visible light in the eye, have been demonstrated in human skin [109, 110] including in melanocytes, which could be modulated by light exposure.

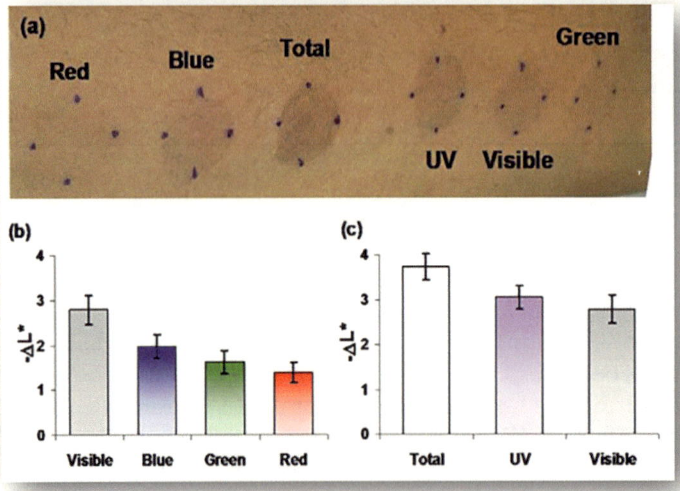

(A)

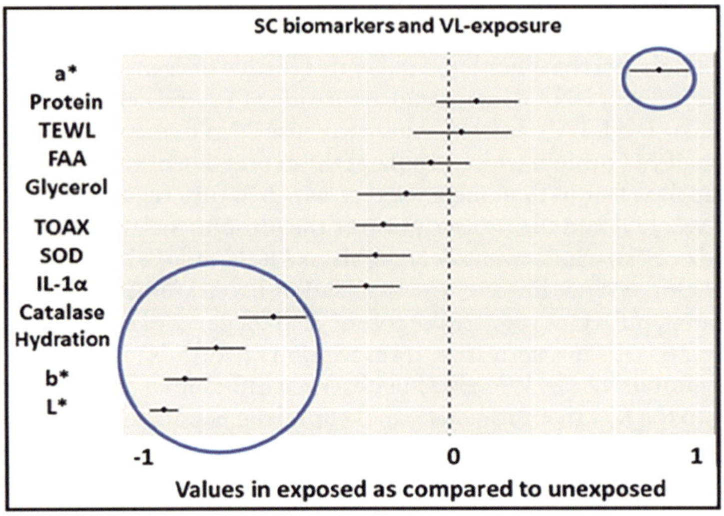

(B)

Figure 2.
Effect of visible light on skin pigmentation—clinical evidence. (A) Effect of different wavelengths of light on skin pigmentation; (B) effect of visible light on color (L, b*, and a*), hydration, TEWL, antioxidants (catalase, total antioxidants [TOAX], superoxide dismutase [SOD], and free fatty acids [faa]), and inflammation markers (IL-1a) as measured from tape strips.*

Multiple studies also suggest that sun exposure (UVA, B, and visible light) could have a role in the induction or exacerbation of hyperpigmentary conditions like freckles, solar lentigines, PIH, melasma, and dark circles [45, 111–113]. In a randomized study with melasma subjects, Castanedo-Cazares et al. [114] showed that UV sunscreens with visible light protection along with 4%HQ treatment significantly improve MASI scores as against just UV protection with HQ treatment [114, 115].

Therefore, it can be assumed that protection is mandatory not only against UV but against the whole spectrum of light as an adjuvant to regular therapy for hyperpigmentation [99, 116]. In addition to UV, the role of blue light /high-energy visible light from non-solar sources like digital devices also needs to be investigated for its contribution to the exacerbation of hyperpigmentation.

4. Cosmetic agents for hyperpigmentation

The consumer desire to achieve uniform skin tone or complexion has been actively supported and promoted by the cosmetic industry for several decades. The commonly used agents for the treatment of hyperpigmentation are hydroquinone, arbutin, kojic acid, and their derivatives, various derivatives of vitamin C, tretinoin, and natural extracts [117] besides chemical peels, lasers, and light-based therapies. This section will focus on topical solutions recommended for hyperpigmentation.

Hydroquinone (HQ) has been the gold standard in the treatment of hyperpigmentation for over five decades although due to its adverse effects (including toxicity and mutagenicity), it is now banned from use in cosmetics or for over-the-counter (OTC) sales in many countries. Currently, HQ is banned in OTC and available only under prescriptions [118, 119], Considering its deleterious effects, consumer interest is shifting to safer and naturally derived actives.

Over time, HQ has been combined with other drugs, with the intent of improving its efficacy. It was Albert Kligman who first developed and demonstrated the efficacy of a formula containing 0.1% tretinoin, 5% hydroquinone, and 0.1% dexamethasone in 1975. A modified Kligman's formula containing 4% HQ, 0.05% tretinoin, and 0.01% fluocinolone acetonide is currently in use, with the backing of successful clinical on melasma patients [120–122]. This mix is popularly called Tri-Luma or the triple combination, can be used across all Fitzpatrick phototypes, and is reported to be better tolerated.

Hydroquinone's action is mostly suggested to be via its ability to inhibit melanin formation by blocking tyrosinase enzyme activity [123, 124]. Deri et al. [125], by visualization studies of HQ in the active site of tyrosinase protein crystals, together with molecular modeling, binding constant analysis, and kinetic experiments, have confirmed that HQ can act both as a tyrosinase enzyme substrate and as an inhibitor. As a substrate, instead of forming melanin, it gets metabolized to quinones and free radicals which cause lipid peroxidation, damaging the melanocyte membrane and leading to melanocyte cytotoxicity and depigmentation [126, 127]. However, in a recent study designed to compare the effects of arbutin, HQ, and kojic acid with numerous resorcinol vis-à-vis inhibition of recombinant human tyrosinase [128, 129], HQ was found to be ineffective against tyrosinase enzyme as compared to resorcinol (**Figure 3**). Thus, although considered to be a tyrosinase inhibitor for a long, it appears that the cytotoxic potential of HQ may largely contribute to its depigmentation effect.

Other tyrosinase inhibitors like arbutin, a derivative of hydroquinone, and kojic acid, have lesser adverse effects, unlike hydroquinone. Glycolic acid, on the other hand, works by causing the desquamation of keratinocytes or epidermolysis when used at higher concentrations [130].

A range of vitamins and their derivatives with enhanced stability or improved dermal penetration are also in use in various cosmetic and pharmaceutical products for skin tone benefits [131, 132].

Vitamin C (VC), also known as ascorbic acid, is a water-soluble vitamin, essential for several processes in human skin, such as dermal collagen synthesis, cell turnover, ROS scavenging, and many more [133]. Emerging evidence indicates that VC and its derivatives can exert therapeutic effects on recalcitrant melasma and facial

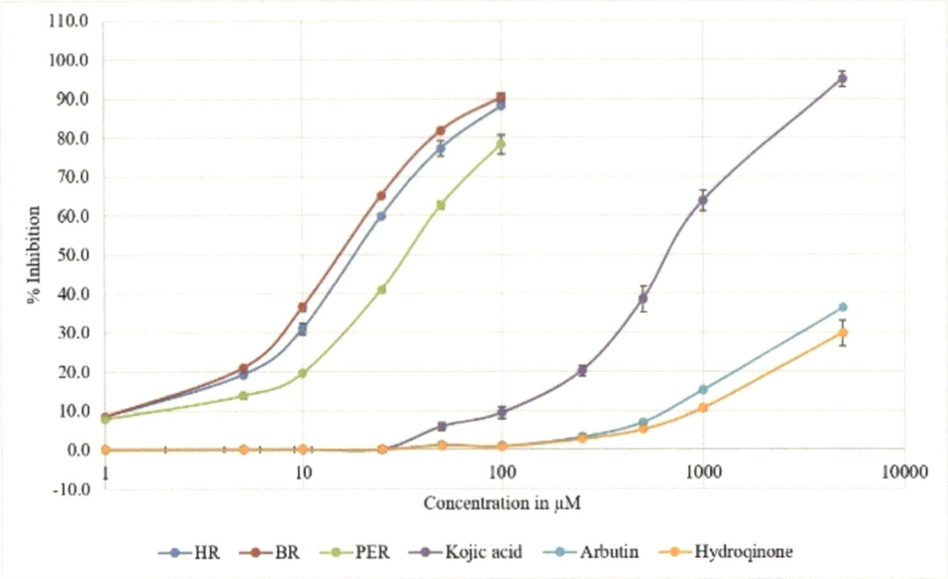

Figure 3.
Inhibition of recombinant human tyrosinase enzyme activity by different resorcinols and known tyrosinase inhibitors. Dose-dependent inhibition of tyrosinase enzyme activity was performed using synthetic recombinant human tyrosinase enzyme protein and DOPA as the substrate.

hyperpigmentation, especially with improved dermal delivery [134, 135]. Vitamin C and its derivatives, magnesium ascorbyl phosphate, and 3-O-ethyl-L-ascorbic acid, exert their depigmenting effect by acidification of the melanocyte cytoplasm, which in turn suppresses the catalytic activity of tyrosinase. Cytoplasmic pH is critical for the catalytic activity of tyrosinase and for the assembly of Pmel17 protein fibrils in the melanosome to form the scaffold upon which melanin is deposited, and any change would therefore influence the melanogenesis process in melanocytes [136, 137]. Vitamin C seems to induce the expression of sodium-dependent VC transporter-2 that further facilitates the transmembrane transport of VC which in turn leads to acidification of the cytoplasm [138]. In addition, 3-O-ethyl-L-ascorbic acid was also shown to modulate the function through *Nrf2*-mediated *α-MSH* inhibition in UVA-irradiated keratinocytes and by autophagy induction and inhibition of *α-MSH*-stimulated melanogenesis in melanocytes [139].

The amide form of vitamin B3, niacinamide has been shown to inhibit melanosome transfer from the melanocytes to the epidermal keratinocytes [140–142]. Various other functions of niacinamide, including improved immunity, barrier function, etc., make it a popular ingredient in multiple cosmetic preparations [132, 143].

Oral and topical tranexamic acid is a recent addition to dermatologists' treatment options to tackle recalcitrant conditions such as melasma and PIH, in combination with other skin tone agents, though more successful studies are needed to back its topical use [144, 145]. In addition, superficial chemical peeling alone or in combination with other topical procedures is also key in the treatment of hyper-pigmentary conditions [146]. In such treatment, avoidance of sun exposure and the use of sunscreens is a must for a successful outcome. Then there are laser and light-based therapies like intense pulsed light, low fluence Q-switched lasers, and non-ablative fractionated lasers that are currently prevalent for use for melasma. Though effective these are also associated with an increased risk of recurrence and PIH [146].

In the next section, we will focus on currently popular cosmetic ingredients such as niacinamide, resorcinol, and retinoids and their potential for the future.

4.1 Niacinamide

Niacinamide has been reported to possess numerous properties, for instance, anti-inflammatory, antimicrobial, immunity booster, bioenergetics modulator, and antioxidant, which makes it suitable for various dermatological uses [132, 143, 147]. Niacinamide can effectively treat various skin conditions viz. aging, hyperpigmentation, acne, rosacea, psoriasis, pruritus, dermatitis, etc. [132, 143]. It increases the biosynthesis of ceramides, as well as other stratum corneum lipids and thus enhances epidermal permeability barrier function [148]. Studies have shown that niacinamide modulated NFkB-mediated inflammatory response, which could support its anti-aging activity [149]. In addition, niacinamide protected against collagen loss in the dermis by preventing its glycation and activation of fibroblast function [150].

Niacinamide is also a well-established and commonly used skin-brightening agent and has been reported to have a significant effect on various hyperpigmentary conditions [142, 151, 152]. Navarrete-Solis et al. [152] showed significant improvement in MASI scores in melasma subjects treated with 4% niacinamide same as for 4% hydroquinone, with less melanin and inflammatory infiltration on histological evaluation of biopsies. However, the lightening effect of hydroquinone was evident as early as the first month of treatment, albeit with some adverse events, whereas with niacinamide, it was noted only in the second month of treatment The effect of niacinamide on melasma was attributed to its anti-inflammatory, melanosome transfer inhibition, and antiaging effects on elastosis [152].

Another study was carried out by a group from Iran [153], on the efficacy of topical 4% niacinamide and 1% clindamycin gels in a randomized, double-blind clinical trial on acne patients with moderate inflammatory acne vulgaris. The mean grade of acne and mean count of papules in patients were comparable in both treatments at the end of the study. In a double-blind study carried out on Indian subjects with acne marks, the application of 1.25% of niacinamide significantly reduced acne marks within 6 weeks as compared to baseline, assessed visually using a skin color scale by an expert dermatologist (**Figure 4A** and **B**) [154].

In an axillary depigmentation trial in phototype III–V, the treatment of 4% niacinamide and desonide 0.05%, significantly reduced the hyperpigmentation of the axillae in 9 weeks versus the placebo group. However, the efficacy of the topical steroid was significantly better than niacinamide treatment and the effect was apparent in desonide-treated subjects by 6 weeks of application. There were also reduced mononuclear and phagocytic cell infiltrates, as well as melanin expression in niacinamide-treated subjects, compared with baseline as determined from the biopsies. However, desonide, in addition, improved the basement membrane as seen in histopathology [155].

Studies have supported the use of anti-inflammatory and depigmenting agents for treatments of PIH, however very few have objectively evaluated PIH development. Damodaran et al. [154] used the sodium dodecyl sulfate (SDS) occluded patch test human trial model of irritation [156] to evaluate the effects of inflammation on pigmentation and the efficacy of niacinamide on inflammation and PIH. The study showed that the pigment or L^* value increased with an increasing irritation score (**Figure 5A**). Pre-application of niacinamide reduced inflammation resulting from SDS and the subsequent development of pigmentation (**Figure 5B** and **C**).

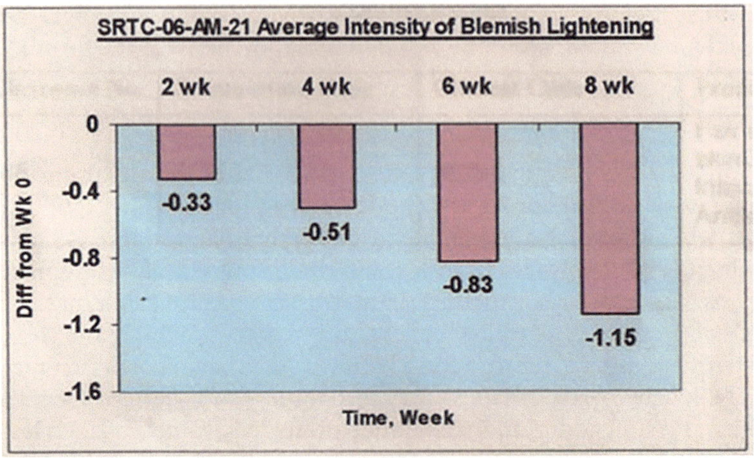

(A)

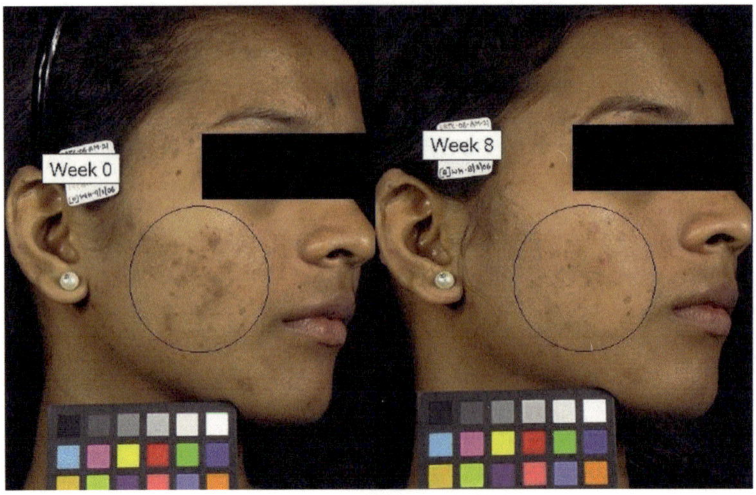

(B)

Figure 4.
Clinical benefits of niacinamide for acne marks. (A) The average extent of lightening of blemishes after product usage for week 2/4/6/8. Statistically significant reduction in the intensity of blemish color at week 2/4/6/8. The negative y-axis values indicate a brightening effect. (B) The facial images of subjects at weeks 0 and 8, after the application of a niacinamide-containing formulation. These photographs are true evidence from the study and are representative of some of the best responders from the study.

A possible molecular mechanism in the efficacy of niacinamide on PIH could be attributed to the modulation of a protein called *SERPINB3* in the skin [157]. Serpin Family B Member 3 (*SERPINB3*) is an endogenous protease inhibitor known for its role in maintaining epidermal barrier homeostasis and is implicated in inflammatory skin conditions including acne [158, 159]. Nair et al. [157] demonstrated that the dermal fibroblasts secrete SERPINB3 in response to inflammatory cytokine interleukin-1 alpha, that in turn induced melanin production in melanocytes (**Figure 6A**). Niacinamide could blunt the *SERPINB3* secretion by fibroblasts (**Figure 6B**) suggesting the novel role of *SERPINB3* in its anti-inflammatory and anti-PIH activity for the potential amelioration of acne and acne marks.

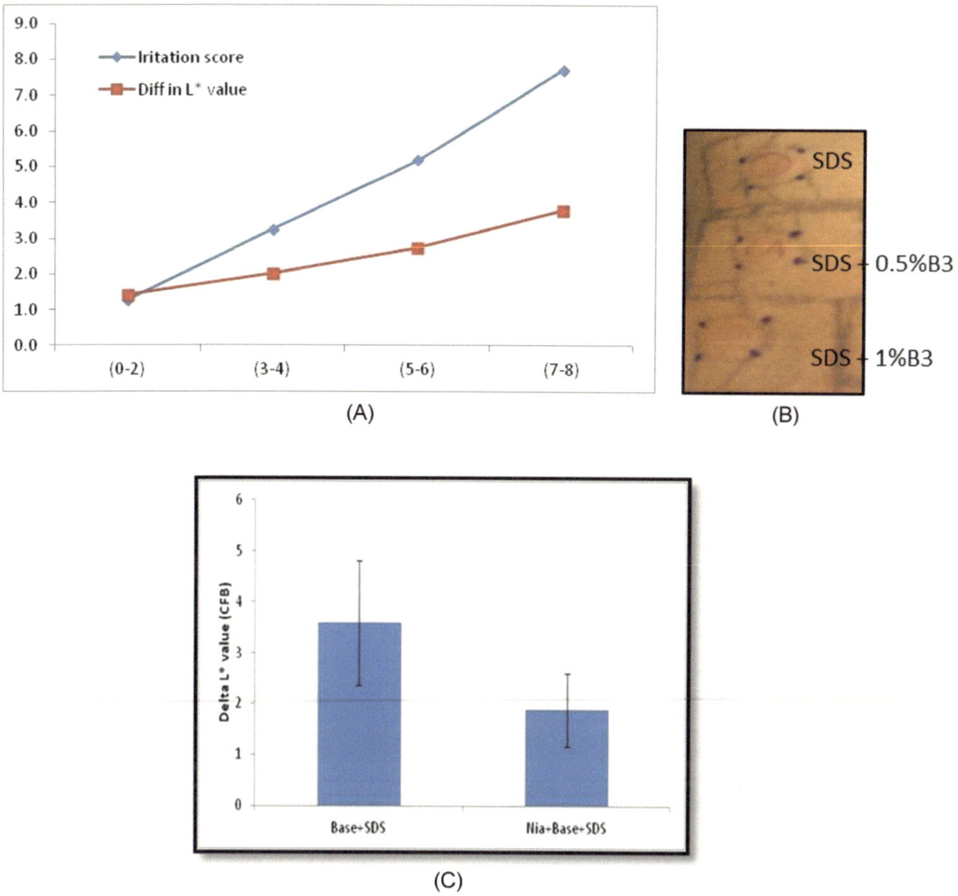

Figure 5.
SDS-induced human occluded patch test. (A) Irritation score induced by SDS follows the trends as with pigmentation (L increase); (B) inhibition of SDS-induced inflammation by pre-application of niacinamide in a dose-dependent manner; (C) niacinamide-containing formulation reduced PIH induced by SDS.*

4.2 Resorcinol

The synthesis and distribution of melanin contribute to skin and hair color in mammals. In human melanocytes, melanin is synthesized within melanosomes by the enzyme tyrosinase, which catalyzes the rate-limiting reaction ie. the conversion of tyrosine to DOPA quinone [160–162].

Tyrosinase, also known as polyphenol oxidase (PPO), is a copper-containing mixed-function oxidase, widely distributed in micro-organisms, animals, and plants. These oxidases catalyze two distinct reactions of melanin synthesis: hydroxylation of a tyrosine a monophenol (monophenolase activity) and the oxidation of DOPA-an o-diphenol to the corresponding o-quinone (diphenolase activity). The quinones formed being highly reactive, polymerize spontaneously to form high molecular weight compounds or pigments—melanin [163]. Melanin is then secreted by melanocyte cells, which are distributed in keratinocytes in the basal layer of the epidermis in the skin. However, abnormal accumulation of melanin has been associated with hyper-pigmentary conditions, including melasma, freckles, and senile lentigines as covered in the earlier section.

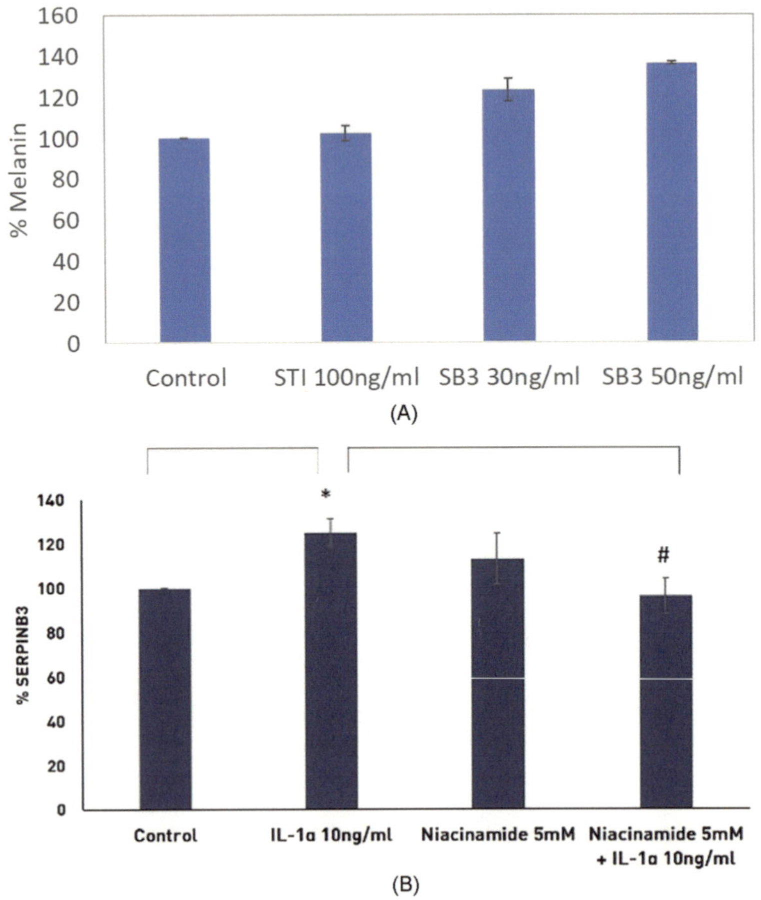

Figure 6.
*Effect of SERPINEB3 on pigmentation and its modulation by niacinamide. (A) 24 h of IL-1α treatment increased SERPINB3 protein secretion (25% vs. control) from dermal fibroblasts. (B) Pre-treatment of cells with 5 mM niacinamide significantly reduced (29% vs. IL-1α) the SERPINB3 secretion of cells. The values are mean ± SE of cells from three independent donors. *p < 0.05 vs. control, #p < 0.05 vs. IL-1α.*

Identification of potent and specific tyrosinase inhibitors has been ongoing for several decades due to its wider implications for the food, pharmaceutical, and cosmetic industries [164, 165]. However, most of the initial discoveries were made using mushroom tyrosinase as a model system [166, 167]. It is only in recent times that more potent tyrosinase inhibitors have been identified using enzymes sourced from human melanocytes or recombinant human tyrosinase protein with superior efficacy on melanotic conditions like solar lentigines and melasma, [129, 168]. The commonly used compounds in the class of tyrosinase inhibitors include hydroquinone, arbutin, kojic acid, thiols, and resorcinol and among them, resorcinol derivatives are the most potent in enzyme inhibition [128, 129]. It has been shown that resorcinol is a mono-oxygenase substrate and gets oxidized to hydroxy intermediate; 3-hydroxy-ortho-quinone, which results in irreversible elimination of Cu (0) of tyrosinase enzyme leading to inactivation of the enzyme [169, 170]. Tyrosinase inhibition activity, though, is mainly attributed to its resorcinol moiety, the efficacy can be further modulated by the various substitution at the 4-position of resorcinol [129, 168, 170]. The levels of tyrosinase inhibition by various 4-resorcinols vary with respect to their alkyl chain length (**Figure 3**).

Phenylethyl resorcinol (PER, 4-(1-phenylethyl)1,3-benzenediol) is a potent inhibitor of tyrosinase [171–173]. PER has been in use as a skin lightener in cosmetics for more than a decade, but the clinical demonstration of its efficacy on hyperpigmentation is limited by its chemical instability to UV light [174, 175].

The clinical efficacy of 4-butyl resorcinol (BR) on the other hand, has been very well established in multiple human trials [173, 176–179]. A randomized, single-blind clinical study was conducted on female subjects with 0.3% 4-butyl resorcinol, 0.3% 4-hexyl resorcinol, and 0.5% 4-phenylethy resorcinol for 12 weeks. 4-butyl resorcinol significantly reduced the appearance of age spots on the forearm after 8 weeks, while others did in 12 weeks. Thereafter, 1% 4-butyl resorcinol was clinically evaluated on age spots on the forearm again; enhancement in skin tone was noticeable by the end of the 16 weeks and was judged to be significant after 4 weeks [173]. The 0.1% 4-butyl resorcinol cream showed rapid efficacy with excellent tolerability in patients with melasma [177, 180]. Liposome-encapsulated 4-butyl resorcinol had a significantly improved effect on the melanin index after 8 weeks of application, without any occurrence of adverse events [178]. In a study on Indian subjects to assess the efficacy, safety, and tolerability of 0.3% 4-butyl resorcinol in melasma patients, a significant decrease in MASI score was observed with no evidence of adverse effect [179].

Another alkyl resorcinol in the skin tone benefit market is 4-hexyl resorcinol (4-HR), an effective tyrosinase inhibitor that was used earlier in the food and medical industries [181–183]. 4-HR has been demonstrated through *in-vitro* and human trials to improve hyperpigmentation through its tyrosinase inhibition activity and its anti-inflammatory potential [184, 185]. 4-HR could regulate collagen and elastin production by inhibiting NF-kB activity in fibroblasts and improving photodamaged skin and clinical signs of aging [186]. Chaudhuri [187] reported multiple benefits of 4-HR, including evidence for its anti-microbial, antioxidant, and anti-glycation effects, along with its effect on extracellular matrix proteins. In a face study by Won et al. [188], 4-HR successfully improved overall skin tone when used in an emulsion over 12 weeks.

The most recent entrant in the skin tone market is the imidazolyl derivative of resorcinol, thiamidol, identified through a high throughput screening of a large compound library on human tyrosinase protein. With an IC50 of 1 μM for tyrosinase enzyme inhibition, it is the most potent inhibitor known so far [129, 168]. The group has also demonstrated the efficacy of thiamidol on various hyperpigmentary conditions like melasma [189–191], solar lentigines [192], PIH [193], and UV-induced skin damage [194] and demonstrated its efficacy to be superior to HQ [190].

The availability of recombinant human tyrosinase protein [128, 129] combined with new platforms that allow for structure-active site prediction based on amino acid sequence [168] will hopefully promote further investigations on tyrosinase chemistry, leading to the identification of inhibitors with greater potency and reduced safety concerns.

In general, as apparent with hydroquinone, the efficacy of a molecule gets compromised when safety becomes paramount. The usage of high doses of ingredients is also a concern in terms of formulation compatibility, sensory, and cost. In such cases, efficacy could be boosted by combining it with other potent agents with a different mode of action and examples do exist where combination therapies have been shown to work for the treatment of recalcitrant hyperpigmentary conditions such as melasma, with a clear example being Kligman's triple combination.

Shariff et al. [128] successfully adopted a combinatorial approach to demonstrate the superior clinical efficacy of a cosmetic formula containing 4-hexyl resorcinol and niacinamide. Based on the in vitro evaluation, appropriate ingredients, and doses were selected to develop a formulation which was then evaluated for spot lightening and anti-aging on Chinese subjects. In the double-blind split-face study comparing 3% niacinamide with 0.4% 4-HR+ 3% niacinamide over 12 weeks of application, significant improvement was achieved for spot lightening and fine lines and wrinkles in crow's feet and perioral areas by the combination of 4HR+ niacinamide over niacinamide alone. This highlighted that combining molecules with different modes of action on pigmentation, resorcinol as a tyrosinase inhibitor and niacinamide as a melanosome transfer and anti-inflammatory molecule, may lead to better and safer skin tone formulas with efficacy on par or better than prescription drugs like hydroquinone.

Another ingredient with a different and established mode of action is retinoid and will be covered in the next section.

4.3 Retinoids

Topical retinoids are recommended by the American academy of dermatology as the first line of treatment for acne and hyperpigmentation, based on strong levels of evidence from well-controlled clinical trials [195, 196]. For issues related to irritation from retinoids, the use of moisturizers is recommended. Dermatologists use tretinoin along with other topical agents and procedures such as superficial chemical peels, to treat hyperpigmentation and improve outcomes [197].

Retinoids have been shown to bind and activate retinoid X nuclear receptors and mediate their cellular function which includes inhibition of keratinocyte proliferation and normalization of follicular differentiation which restores normal desquamation and helps to unclog pores [198]. Retinoids are also anti-inflammatory and suppress toll-like receptors, cytokine, and nitric oxide production [199, 200]. It also corrects pigmentation by inhibiting melanosome transfer and the rate of epidermal turnover [196].

Though tretinoin is recommended for the treatment of dark circles [201], melasma [202], and acne [203], some new retinoid derivatives such as adapalene, tazarotene, and trifarotene have also come into the market for dermatological usage [204, 205].

The effects of retinoids on hyperpigmentation have been evaluated in various studies, either for efficacy or safety assessment, with favorable results [195]. Tretinoin was the first retinoid specifically evaluated on hyperpigmentation in patients with melanin-rich skin. Tretinoin reduced hyperpigmented lesions mostly due to PIH in phototype IV–VI skin subjects, with improvement evident as early as week 4 [206]. However, irritation continued to be an issue and was managed by emollients and moisturizers.

The new derivative, tazarotene has FDA approval at 0.1% levels for use as an adjunct for the treatment of fine lines and wrinkles, mottled hyperpigmentation, and lentigines on the face [207]. In an acne-induced PIH or marks study with skin types III-VI, statistically significant reductions were achieved with tazarotene versus vehicle on hyperpigmented lesions, [208]. However, adverse events were still observed with tazarotene as in the case of tretinoin. Trifarotene 0.005% cream is a fourth-generation retinoid approved for the treatment of facial and truncal acne [209], but its clinical effects on PIH in patients with skin of color have not yet been reported.

Combination therapies are the mainstay of retinoid therapies which also help counteract associated irritation issues, essentially either with other topical drugs like HQ, clindamycin or light/laser therapies [196, 197].

Retinyl esters, such as retinyl propionate, are known to be less irritating and less efficacious than retinol or tretinoin and this was hypothesized to be the result of rapid degradation of retinoic acid generated endogenously from esters, by P450 (CYP) protein. Adamus et al. [210] demonstrated the use of climbazole a weak pan-inhibitor P450 (CYP) to prevent loss due to the degradation of retinoic acid thus boosting the efficacy of retinyl propionate in vitro. This was followed by a human trial which confirmed the hypothesis and demonstrated that retinyl propionate alone, and in combination with climbazole, was significantly less irritating than a similar serum containing retinol. The retinyl propionate with climbazole serum treatment also showed equal, or better efficacy than retinol alone serum on fine and coarse lines and wrinkles, as well as pigmentation. Additionally, the combined retinol/climbazole was shown to modulate histological biomarkers of skin aging viz. epidermal thickness, procollagen-1 protein, Ki-67, and retinoid activity (CRABP2, KRT4) [211].

Thus, milder but efficacious retinoids like retinyl propionate with climbazole could be another ingredient with a different mode of activity for the exploration of potential combinations in the future.

5. Conclusion

Melanin in the skin provides better photoprotection to melanated skin. However, abnormal accumulation of melanin as seen in hyperpigmentary conditions, *viz.* melasma, freckles, senile lentigines, etc. is undesirable. Hyperpigmentary conditions are by and large refractory and recurrent in nature, particularly to traditional cosmetic actives. Multiple risk factors, together with the complex and less understood biology of these conditions, largely contribute to poor treatment outcomes. The most effective interventions for their management are mostly drug-based preparations and physical methods such as lasers that are not very well tolerated, particularly in skin of color.

A comprehensive understanding of hyperpigmentation biology combined with the development of potent mixes that target multiple pathogenic mechanisms is likely the way to provide prescription strength efficacy for its control, without associated safety concerns and side effects. Also, as our understanding of the impact of sunlight and its various components (besides UV) on skin pigmentation and health improves, it is imperative to educate consumers on the diligent use of more comprehensive sun protection measures, regardless of skin phototype.

Author details

Anita Damodaran* and Nirmala Nair
Unilever R&D, Bangalore, India

*Address all correspondence to: anita.damodaran@unilever.com

References

[1] Pavan WJ, Strum RA. The genetics of human skin and hair pigmentation. Annual Review of Genomics and Human Genetics. 2019;**20**:41-72. DOI: 10.1146/annurev-genom-083118-015230

[2] Naik PP, Farrukh SN. Influence of ethnicities and skin color variations in different populations: A review. Skin Pharmacology and Physiology. 2022;**35**:65-76. DOI: 10.1159/000518826

[3] Deng L, Xu S. Adaptation of human skin color in various populations. Hereditas. 2018;**155**:1-12. DOI: 10.1186/s41065-017-0036-2

[4] Martin AR, Lin M, Granka JM, Myrick JW, Liu X, Sockell A, et al. An unexpectedly complex architecture for skin pigmentation in Africans. Cell. 2017;**171**:1340-1353. DOI: 10.1016/j.cell.2017.11.015

[5] Nip J, Potterf B, Rocha S, Vora S, Bosko C. The new face of pigmentation and aging. In: Farage MA, Miller KW, Maibach HI, editors. Textbook of Aging Skin. Springer Publishers; 2010. pp. 1039-1054. DOI: 10.1007/978-3-662-47398-6_53

[6] Bastiaens MT, Westendorp RG, Vermeer BJ, Bavinck JN. Ephelides are more related to pigmentary constitutional host factors than solar lentigines. Pigment Cell Research. 1999;**12**:316-322. DOI: 10.1111/j.1600-0749

[7] Bastiaens MT, Hoefnagel J, Westendorp R, Vermeer BJ, Bavinck JN. Solar lentigines are strongly related to sun exposure in contrast to ephelides. Pigment Cell Research. 2004;**17**:225-229. DOI: 10.1111/j.1600-0749.2004.00131.x

[8] Rahman SB, Bhawan J. Lentigo. International Journal of Dermatology. 1996;**35**:229-239. DOI: 10.1111/j.1365-4362.1996.tb02994.x

[9] Nakamura M, Morita A, Seite S, Stemmann TH, Beck SG, Krutmann J. Environment-induced lentigines: Formation of solar lentigines beyond ultraviolet radiation. Experimental Dermatology. 2015;**24**:407-411. DOI: 10.1111/exd.12690

[10] Andersen WK, Labadie RR, Bhawan J. Histopathology of solar lentigines of the face: A quantitative study. Journal of the American Academy of Dermatology. 1997;**36**:444-447. DOI: 10.1016/s0190-9622(97)80224-1

[11] Yonei N, Kaminaka C, Kimura A, Furukawa F, Yamamoto Y. Two patterns of solar lentigines: A histopathological analysis of 40 Japanese women. The Journal of Dermatology. 2012;**39**:829-832. DOI: 10.1111/j.1346-8138.2012.01574.x

[12] Lin CB, Hu Y, Rossetti D, Chen N, David C, Slominski A, et al. Immunohistochemical evaluation of solar lentigines: The association of KGF/KGFR and other factors with lesion development. Journal of Dermatological Science. 2010;**59**:91-97. DOI: 10.1016/j.jdermsci.2010.06.006

[13] Cario-Andre M, Lepreux S, Pain C, Nizard C, Noblesse E, Taieb A. Perilesional vs. lesional skin changes in senile lentigo. Journal of Cutaneous Pathology. 2004;**31**:441-447. DOI: 10.1111/j.0303-6987.2004.00210.x

[14] Aoki H, Moro O, Tagami H, Kishimoto J. Gene expression profiling analysis of solar lentigo in relation to immunohistochemical characteristics. The British Journal of Dermatology. 2007;**156**:1214-1223. DOI: 10.1111/j.1365-2133.2007.07830.x

[15] Jung JM, Yang H, Lee WJ, Won CH, Lee MW, Choi JH, et al. Inflammatory features and rete ridge patterns of facial solar lentigo may guide laser treatment. Dermatologic Therapy. 2020;**33**:e13464. DOI: 10.1111/dth.13464

[16] Hafner C, Stoehr R, van Oers JM, Zwarthoff EC, Hofstaedter F, Landthaler M, et al. FGFR3 and PIK3CA mutations are involved in the molecular pathogenesis of solar lentigo. The British Journal of Dermatology. 2009;**160**:546-551. DOI: 10.1111/j.1365-2133.2008.08963.x

[17] Choi W, Yin L, Smuda C, Batzer J, Hearing VJ, Kolbe L. Molecular and histological characterization of age spots. Dermatologica. 2017;**26**:242-248. DOI: 10.1111/exd.13203

[18] Ganesh C, Damodaran A, Green MR, Rocha S, Pauloski N, Vora S. Multiple genes and diverse hierarchical pathways affect human pigmentation. In: Smith J, Haworth M, editors. Skin Pigmentation. Nova Science Publishers; 2013. pp. 89-119

[19] Shin J, Park JY, Kim SJ, Kang HY. Characteristics of keratinocytes in facial solar lentigo with flattened rete ridges: Comparison with melasma. Clinical and Experimental Dermatology. 2015;**40**:489-494. DOI: 10.1111/ced.12621

[20] Barysch MJ, Braun RP, Kolm I, Ahlgrimm-Siesz V, Hofmann-Wellenhof R, Duval C, et al. Keratinocytic malfunction as a trigger for the development of solar lentigines. Dermatopathology (Basel). 2019;**6**:1-11. DOI: 10.1159/000495404

[21] Kovacs D, Cardinali G, Aspite N, Cota C, Luzi F, Bellei B, et al. Role of fibroblast-derived growth factors in regulating hyperpigmentation of solar lentigo. The British Journal of Dermatology. 2010;**163**:1020-1027. DOI: 10.1111/j.1365-2133.2010.09946.x

[22] Goorochurn R, Viennet C, Tissot M, Locatelli F, Granger C, Varin-Blank N, et al. Differential morphological and functional features of fibroblasts explanted from solar lentigo. The British Journal of Dermatology. 2017;**1177**:109-e111. DOI: 10.1111/bjd.15386

[23] Imokawa G. Melanocyte activation mechanisms and rational therapeutic treatments of solar lentigos. International Journal of Molecular Sciences. 2019;**20**:3666. DOI: 10.3390/ijms20153666

[24] Iriyama S, Ono T, Aoki H, Amano S. Hyperpigmentation in human solar lentigo is promoted by heparanase-induced loss of heparan sulfate chains at the dermal-epidermal junction. Journal of Dermatological Science. 2011;**64**:223-228. DOI: 10.1016/j.jdermsci.2011.09.007

[25] Hasegawa K, Fujiwara R, Sato K, Park JY, Kim SJ, Kim M, et al. Increased blood flow and vasculature in solar lentigo. The Journal of Dermatology. 2016;**43**:1209-1213. DOI: 10.1111/1346-8138.13458

[26] Shibata T, Kajiya K, Sato K, Yoon J, Kang HY. 3D microvascular analysis reveals irregularly branching blood vessels in the hyperpigmented skin of solar lentigo. Pigment Cell & Melanoma Research. 2018;**31**:725-727. DOI: 10.1111/pcmr.12731

[27] Hara Y, Yamashita T, Ninomiya M, Kubo Y, Katagiri C, Saeki S, et al. Vascular morphology in facial solar lentigo assessed by optical coherence tomography angiography. Journal of Dermatological Science. 2021;**102**:193-195. DOI: 10.1016/j.jdermsci.2021.04.001

[28] Kerns ML, Chien AL, Kang S. A role for NRF2-signaling in the treatment and prevention of solar lentigines. Plastic and Reconstructive Surgery.

2021;**148**:27S-31S. DOI: 10.1097/PRS.0000000000008783

[29] Epstein JH. Postinflammatory hyperpigmentation. Clinics in Dermatology. 1989;**7**:55-65. DOI: 10.1016/0738-081x(89)90057-6

[30] Taylor S, Grimes P, Lim J, Im S, Lui H. Postinflammatory hyperpigmentation. Journal of Cutaneous Medicine and Surgery. 2009;**13**:183-191. DOI: 10.2310/7750.2009.08077

[31] Perkins AC, Cheng CE, Hillebrand GG, Miyamoto K, Kimball AB. Comparison of the epidemiology of acne vulgaris among Caucasian, Asian, Continental Indian and African American women. Journal of the European Academy of Dermatology and Venereology. 2011;**25**:1054-1060. DOI: 10.1111/j.1468-3083.2010.03919.x

[32] Ruiz-Maldonado R, Orozco-Covarrubias ML. Postinflammatory hypopigmentation and hyperpigmentation. Seminars in Cutaneous Medicine and Surgery. 1997;**16**:36-43. DOI: 10.1016/s1085-5629(97)80034-x

[33] Silpa-Archa N, Kohli I, Chaowattanapanit S, Lim HW, Hamzavi I. Postinflammatory hyperpigmentation: A comprehensive overview: Epidemiology, pathogenesis, clinical presentation, and non-invasive assessment technique. Journal of the American Academy of Dermatology. 2017;**77**:591-605. DOI: 10.1016/j.jaad.2017.01.035

[34] Lacz NL, Vafaie J, Kihiczak NI, Schwartz RA. Postinflammatory hyperpigmentation: A common but troubling condition. International Journal of Dermatology. 2004;**3**:362-365. DOI: 10.1111/j.1365-4632.2004.02267.x

[35] Alster TS, Nanni CA, Williams CM. Comparison of four carbon dioxide resurfacing lasers: A clinical and histopathologic evaluation. Dermatologic Surgery. 1999;**25**:153-159. DOI: 10.1046/j.1524-4725.1999.08126.x

[36] Bernstein LJ, Kauvar ANB, Grossman MC, Geronemus RG. The short- and long-term side effects of carbon dioxide laser resurfacing. Dermatologic Surgery. 1997;**23**:519-525. DOI: 10.1111/j.1524-4725.1997.tb00677.x

[37] Harari Z, Sommer I, Knobel B. Multifocal contact dermatitis to nitroderm TTS 5 with extensive postinflammatory hypermelanosis. Dermatologica. 1987;**174**:249-252. DOI: 10.1159/000249190

[38] Abad-Casintahan F, Chow SK, Goh CL, Kubba R, Hayashi N, Noppakun N, et al. Frequency and characteristics of acne-related post-inflammatory hyperpigmentation. Asian Acne Board. Journal of Dermatology. 2016;**3**:826-828. DOI: 10.1111/1346-8138.13263

[39] Evans RL, Marriott RE, Harker M. Axillary skin: Biology and care. International Journal of Cosmetic Science. 2012;**34**:389-395. DOI: 10.1111/j.1468-2494.2012.00729.x

[40] Park JY, Park JH, Kim SJ, Kwon JE, Kang HY, Lee ES, et al. Two histopathological patterns of postinflammatory hyperpigmentation: Epidermal and dermal. Journal of Cutaneous Pathology. 2017;**44**:118-124. DOI: 10.1111/cup.12849

[41] Masu S, Seiji M. Pigmentary incontinence in fixed drug eruptions. Histologic and electron microscopic findings. Journal of the American Academy of Dermatology. 1983;**8**:525-532. DOI: 10.1016/s0190-9622(83)70060-5

[42] Maghfour J, Olayinka J, Hamzavi IH, Mohammad TF. A focused review on the pathophysiology of post-inflammatory hyperpigmentation. Pigment Cell & Melanoma Research. 2022;**35**:320-327. DOI: 10.1111/pcmr.13038

[43] Roh MR, Chung KY. Infraobital dark circles: Definition, causes, and treatment options. Dermatologic Surgery. 2009;**35**:1163-1171. DOI: 10.1111/j.1524-4725.2009.01213.x

[44] Grimes PE. Aesthetics and Cosmetic Surgery for Darker Skin Types. 1st ed. Lippincott Williams & Wilkins (LWW); 2007

[45] Sheth PB, Shah HA, Dave JN. Periorbital hyperpigmentation: A study of its prevalence, common causative factors and its association with personal habits and other disorders. Indian Journal of Dermatology. 2014;**59**:151-157. DOI: 10.4103/0019-5154.127675

[46] Freitag FM, Cestari TF. What causes dark circles under the eyes? Journal of Cosmetic Dermatology. 2007;**6**:211-215. DOI: 10.1111/j.1473-2165.2007.00324.x

[47] Sardana K, Rajpal M, Garg V, Mishra D. Periorbital hyperpigmentation mimicking fixed drug eruption: A rare presentation of erythema dyschromicum perstans in a paediatric patient. Journal of the European Academy of Dermatology and Venereology. 2006;**20**:1381-1383. DOI: 10.1111/j.1468-3083.2006.01735.x

[48] Lim HGY, Fischer AH, Sung S, Kang S, Al C. Periocular dark circles: Correlates of severity. Annals of Dermatology. 2021;**33**:393-401. DOI: 10.5021/ad.2021.33.5.393

[49] Goldberg RA, McCann JD, Fiaschetti D, Simon GJ. What causes eyelid bags? Analysis of 114 consecutive patients. Plastic and Reconstructive Surgery. 2005;**115**:1395-1402. DOI: 10.1097/01.prs.0000157016.49072.61

[50] Sawant O, Khan T. Management of periorbital hyperpigmentation: An overview of nature-based agents and alternative approaches. Dermatologic Therapy. 2020;**33**:e13717. DOI: 10.1111/dth.13717

[51] Ranu H, Thng S, Goh BK, Burger A, Goh CL. Periorbital hyperpigmentation in Asians: An epidemiologic study and a proposed classification. Dermatologic Surgery. 2011;**37**:1297-1303. DOI: 10.1111/j.1524-4725.2011.02065.x

[52] Sarkar R, Ranjan R, Garg S, Garg VK, Sonthalia S, Bansal S. Periorbital hyperpigmentation: A comprehensive review. The Journal of Clinical and Aesthetic Dermatology. 2016;**9**:49-55

[53] Sarkar R, Das A. Periorbital hyperpigmentation: What lies beneath? Indian Dermatology Online Journal. 2018;**9**:229-230. DOI: 10.4103/idoj.IDOJ_303_17

[54] Daroach M, Kumaran MS. Periorbital hyperpigmentation – An overview of the enigmatous condition. Pigment International. 2018;**5**:1-3

[55] Nouveau S, Agrawal D, Kohli M, Bernerd F, Misra N. Skin hyperpigmentation in Indian population: Insights and best practice. Indian Journal of Dermatology. 2016;**61**:487-495. DOI: 10.4103/0019-5154.190103

[56] Grimes PE, Ijaz S, Nashawati R, Kwak D. New oral and topical approaches for the treatment of melasma. International Journal of Women's Dermatology. 2019;**5**:30-36. DOI: 10.1016/j.ijwd.2018.09.004

[57] Watanabe S, Nakai K, Ohnishi T. Condition known as "dark rings under the eyes" in the Japanese population is a kind of dermal melanocytosis which can be successfully treated by Q-switched ruby laser. Dermatologic Surgery. 2006;**32**:785-789. DOI: 10.1111/j.1524-4725.2006.32161.x

[58] Graziosi AC, Quaresma MR, Michalany NS, Ferreira LM. Cutaneous idiopathic hyperchromia of the orbital region (CIHOR): A histopathological study. Aesthetic Plastic Surgery. 2013;**37**:434-438. DOI: 10.1007/s00266-012-0048-2

[59] Kurita M, Kato H, Yoshimura K. A therapeutic strategy based on histological assessment of hyperpigmented skin lesions in Asians. Journal of Plastic, Reconstructive & Aesthetic Surgery. 2009;**62**:955-963. DOI: 10.1016/j.bjps.2007.10.079

[60] Mac-Mary S, Solinis IZ, Predine O, Sainthillier JM, Sladen C, Bell M, et al. Identification of three key factors contributing to the aetiology of dark circles by clinical and instrumental assessments of the infraorbital region. Clinical, Cosmetic and Investigational Dermatology. 2019;**18**:919-929. DOI: 10.2147/CCID.S217956

[61] Perez BA, Perez MA, Camacho F. Management of facial hyperpigmentation. American Journal of Clinical Dermatology. 2000;**1**:261-268. DOI:10.2165/00128071-200001050-00001

[62] Sheth VM, Pandya AG. Melasma: A comprehensive update Part 1. Journal of the American Academy of Dermatology. 2011;**65**:689-697. DOI: 10.1016/j.jaad.2010.12.046

[63] Grimes PE. Melasma: Etiologic and therapeutic considerations. Archives of Dermatology. 1995;**131**:1453-1457. DOI: 10.1001/archderm.131.12.1453

[64] Passeron T, Picardo M. Melasma, a photoaging disorder. Pigment Cell & Melanoma Research. 2018;**31**(4):461-465. DOI: 10.1111/pcmr.12684

[65] Ortonne JP, Arellano I, Berneburg M, Cestari T, Chan H, Grimes P, et al. A global survey of the role of ultraviolet radiation and hormonal influences in the development of melasma. Journal of the European Academy of Dermatology and Venereology. 2009;**23**:1254-1262. DOI: 10.1111/j.1468-3083.2009.03295.x

[66] Handel AC, Miot LD, Miot HA. Melasma: A clinical and epidemiological review. Anais Brasileiros de Dermatologia. 2014;**89**:771-782. DOI: 10.1590/abd1806-4841.20143063

[67] Khanna N, Rasool S. Facial melanoses: Indian perspective. Indian Journal of Dermatology, Venereology and Leprology. 2011;**77**:552. DOI: 10.4103/0378-6323.84046

[68] Lee AY. Recent progress in melasma pathogenesis. Pigment Cell & Melanoma Research. 2015;**28**:648-660. DOI: 10.1111/pcmr.12404

[69] Suryaningsih BE, Sadewa AH, Wirohadidjojo YW, Soebono H. Association between heterozygote Val92Met MC1R gene polymorphisms with incidence of melasma: A study of Javanese women population in Yogyakarta. Clinical, Cosmetic and Investigational Dermatology. 2019;**12**:489-495. DOI: 10.2147/CCID.S206115

[70] Kheradmand M, Afshari M, Damiani G, Abediankenari S, Moosazadeh M. Melasma and thyroid disorders: A systematic review and meta-analysis. International Journal of Dermatology. 2019;**58**:1231-1238. DOI: 10.1111/ijd.14497

[71] Artzi O, Horovitz T, Bar-Ilan E, Shehadeh W, Koren A, Zusmanovitch L,

et al. The pathogenesis of melasma and implications for treatment. Journal of Cosmetic Dermatology. 2021;**20**:3432-3445. DOI: 10.1111/jocd.14382

[72] Kang HY, Suzuki I, Lee DJ, Ha J, Reiniche P, Aubert J, et al. Transcriptional profiling shows altered expression of WNT pathway- and lipid metabolism-related genes as well as melanogenesis-related genes in melasma. The Journal of Investigative Dermatology. 2011;**131**:1692-1700. DOI: 10.1038/jid.2011.109

[73] Kim JY, Lee TR, Lee AY. Reduced WIF-1 expression stimulates skin hyperpigmentation in patients with melasma. The Journal of Investigative Dermatology. 2013;**133**:191-200. DOI: 10.1038/jid.2012.270

[74] Jang YH, Lee JY, Kang HY, Lee ES, Kim YC. Oestrogen and progesterone receptor expression in melasma: An immunohistochemical analysis. Journal of the European Academy of Dermatology and Venereology. 2010;**24**:1312-1316. DOI: 10.1111/j.1468-3083.2010.03638.x

[75] Tamega Ade A, Miot HA, Moc ONP, Silva MG, Marques ME, Miot LD. Gene and protein expression of oestrogen-b and progesterone receptors in facial melasma and adjacent healthy skin in women. International Journal of Cosmetic Science. 2015;**37**:222-228. DOI: 10.1111/ics.12186

[76] Kim NH, Cheong KA, Lee TR, Lee AY. PDZK1 upregulation in estrogen-related hyperpigmentation in melasma. The Journal of Investigative Dermatology. 2012;**132**:2622-2631. DOI: 10.1038/jid.2012.175

[77] Kim EH, Kim YC, Lee ES, Kang HY. The vascular characteristics of melasma. Journal of Dermatological Science. 2007;**46**:111-116. DOI: 10.1016/j.jdermsci.2007.01.009

[78] Kang HY, Bahadoran P, Suzuki I, Zugaj D, Khemis A, Passeron T, et al. In vivo reflectance confocal microscopy detects pigmentary changes in melasma at a cellular level resolution. Experimental Dermatology. 2010;**19**:e228-e233. DOI: 10.1111/j.1600-0625.2009.01057.x

[79] Passeron T. Long-lasting effect of vascular targeted therapy of melasma. Journal of the American Academy of Dermatology. 2013;**69**:e141-e142. DOI: 10.1016/j.jaad.2013.02.022

[80] Jo HY, Kim CK, Suh IB, Ryu SW, Ha KS, Kwon YG, et al. Co-localization of inducible nitric oxide synthase and phosphorylated Akt in the lesional skins of patients with melasma. The Journal of Dermatology. 2009;**36**:10-16. DOI: 10.1111/j.1346-8138.2008.00579.x

[81] Kang HY, Hwang JS, Lee JY, Ahn JH, Kim JY, Lee ES, et al. The dermal stem cell factor and c-kit are overexpressed in melasma. The British Journal of Dermatology. 2006;**154**:1094-1099. DOI: 10.1111/j.1365-2133.2006.07179.x

[82] Regazzetti C, De Donatis GM, GhorbelHH,Cardot-LecciaN,AmbrosettiD, Bahadoran P, et al. Endothelial cells promote pigmentation through Endothelin Receptor B activation. The Journal of Investigative Dermatology. 2015;**135**:3096. DOI: 10.1038/jid.2015.332

[83] Hernandez-Barrera R, Torres-Alvarez B, Castanedo-Cazares JP, Oros-Ovalle C, Moncada B. Solar elastosis and presence of mast cells as key features in the pathogenesis of melasma. Clinical and Experimental Dermatology. 2008;**33**:305-308. DOI: 10.1111/j.1365-2230.2008.02724. x

[84] Torres-Álvarez B, Mesa-Garza IG, Castanedo-Cázares JP, Fuentes-Ahumada C, Oros-Ovalle C, Navarrete-Solis J, et al. Histochemical and immunohistochemical study in melasma: Evidence of damage in the basal membrane. The American Journal of Dermatopathology. 2011;**33**:291-295. DOI: 10.1097/DAD.0b013e3181ef2d45

[85] Iddamalgoda A, Le QT, Ito K, Tanaka K, Kojima H, Kido H. Mast cell tryptase and photoaging: Possible involvement in the degradation of extra cellular matrix and basement membrane proteins. Archives of Dermatological Research. 2008;**300**(Suppl. 1):S69-S76. DOI: 10.1007/s00403-007-0806-1

[86] Lee DJ, Park KC, Ortonne JP, Kang HY. Pendulous melanocytes: A characteristic feature of melasma and how it may occur. The British Journal of Dermatology. 2012;**166**:684-686. DOI: 10.1111/j.1365-2133.2011.10648.x

[87] Inomata S, Matsunaga Y, Amano S, Takada K, Kobayashi K, Tsunenaga M, et al. Possible involvement of gelatinases in basement membrane damage and wrinkle formation in chronically ultraviolet B-exposed hairless mouse. The Journal of Investigative Dermatology. 2003;**120**:128-134. DOI: 10.1046/j.1523-1747.2003.12021.x

[88] Kang WH, Yoon KH, Lee ES, Kim J, Lee KB, Yim H, et al. Melasma: Histopathological characteristics in 56 Korean patients. The British Journal of Dermatology. 2002;**146**:228-237. DOI: 10.1046/j.0007-0963.2001.04556.x

[89] Lentsch G, Balu M, Williams J, Lee S, Harris R, König K, et al. In vivo multiphoton microscopy of melasma. Pigment Cell & Melanoma Research. 2019;**32**:403-411. DOI: 10.1111/pcmr.12756

[90] Christensen L, Suggs A, Baron E. Ultraviolet photobiology in dermatology. Advances in Experimental Medicine and Biology. 2017;**996**:89-104. DOI: 10.1007/978-3-319-56017-5_8

[91] Kohli I, Sakamaki T, Tian WD, Moyal D, Hamzavi IH, Kollias N. The dynamics of pigment reactions of human skin to ultraviolet A radiation. Photodermatology, Photoimmunology & Photomedicine. 2019;**35**:387-392. DOI: 10.1111/phpp.12497

[92] Mahmoud BH, Ruvolo E, Hexsel CL, Liu Y, Owen MR, Kollias N, et al. Impact of long-wavelength UVA and visible light on melanocompetent skin. The Journal of Investigative Dermatology. 2010;**130**:2092-2097. DOI: 10.1038/jid.2010.95

[93] Amaro-Ortiz A, Yan B, D'Orazio JA. Ultraviolet radiation, aging, and the skin: Prevention of damage by topical cAMP manipulation. Molecules. 2014;**19**:6202-6219. DOI: 10.3390/molecules19056202

[94] Cadet J, Douki T. Formation of UV-induced DNA damage contributing to skin cancer development. Photochemical & Photobiological Sciences. 2018;**17**:1816-1841. DOI: 10.1039/c7pp00395a

[95] Box NF, Terzian T. The role of p53 in pigmentation, tanning and melanoma. Pigment Cell & Melanoma Research. 2008;**21**:525-533. DOI: 10.1111/j.1755-148X.2008.00495.x

[96] Cui R, Widlund HR, Feige E, Lin JY, Wilensky DL, Igras VE, et al. Central role of p53 in the suntan response and pathologic hyperpigmentation. Cell. 2007;**128**:853-864. DOI: 10.1016/j.cell.2006.12.045

[97] Paik SH, Kim H-J, Son H-Y, Lee S, Im S-W, Ju YS, et al. Gene mapping study

for constitutive skin color in an isolated Mongolian population. Experimental & Molecular Medicine. 2012;**44**:241-249. DOI: 10.3858/emm.2012.44.3.020

[98] Austin E, Geisler AN, Nguyen J, Kohli I, Hamzavi I, Lim HW, et al. Part I: Properties and cutaneous effects of visible light. Journal of the American Academy of Dermatology. 2022;**84**:1219-1231. DOI: 10.1016/j.jaad.2021.02.048

[99] Lim HW, Kohli I, Ruvolo E, Kolbe L, Hamzavi IH. Impact of visible light on skin health: The role of antioxidants and free radical quenchers in skin protection. Journal of the American Academy of Dermatology. 2022;**86**(3S):S27-S37. DOI: 10.1016/j.jaad.2021.12.024

[100] Ramasubramaniam R, Roy A, Sharma B, Nagalakshmi S. Are there mechanistic differences between ultraviolet and visible radiation induced skin pigmentation? Photochemical & Photobiological Sciences. 2011;**10**:1887-1893. DOI: 10.1039/c1pp05202k

[101] Gosh Dastidar S, Rajkumar S, Rajgopal R, and Damodaran A. Impact of high energy visible light on skin appearance. Journal of the American Academy of Dermatology. 2018;**79**(3): AB159. DOI: https://doi.org/10.1016/j.jaad.2018.05.653. Annual meeting of American Academy of Dermatology (AAD), 16-20 February 2018, San Diego, California, USA

[102] Kim S, Rainer BM, Qi J, Brown I, Ogurtsova A, Leung S, et al. Clinical and molecular change induced by repeated low-dose visible light exposure in both light-skinned and dark-skinned individuals. Photodermatology, Photoimmunology & Photomedicine. 2022:1-9. DOI: 10.1111/phpp.12819

[103] Moreiras H, O'Connor C, Bell M, Tobin DJ. Visible light and human skin pigmentation: The importance of skin phototype. Experimental Dermatology. 2021;**30**:1324-1331. DOI: 10.1111/exd.14400

[104] Liebel F, Kaur S, Ruvolo E, Kollias N, Southall MD. Irradiation of skin with visible light induces reactive oxygen species and matrix-degrading enzymes. The Journal of Investigative Dermatology. 2012;**132**:1901-1907. DOI: 10.1038/jid.2011.476

[105] Rajkumar S, Roy A, Surendra N, Gupta AK, Joshi M, and Damodaran A. Visible light effects on skin function and pigmentation. In: 8th annual meeting of ASPCR, 12-13 November 2016, Kaohsiung, Taiwan

[106] Damodaran A, Rajkumar S, Shruthi PB, Patil N, Kumar S, and Kale V. Novel role of visible and blue light in modulation of inflammation and molecular clock genes in skin cells, in vitro. In: 24th World Congress of Dermatology; 10-15 June 2019, Milan, Italy

[107] Campiche R, Curpen SJ, Lutchmanen-Kolanthan V, Gougeon S, Cherel M, Laurent G, et al. Pigmentation effects of blue light irradiation on skin and how to protect against them. International Journal of Cosmetic Science. 2020;**42**:399-406. DOI: 10.1111/ics.12367

[108] Zhao Z, Zhou Y, Tan G, Li J. Research progress about the effect and prevention of blue light on eyes. International Journal of Ophthalmology. 2018;**11**:1999-2003. DOI: 10.18240/ijo.2018.12.20

[109] Suh S, Choi EH, Mesinkovska NA. The expression of opsins in the human skin and its implications for photobiomodulation: A systematic review. Photodermatology,

Photoimmunology & Photomedicine. 2020;**36**:329-338. DOI: 10.1111/phpp.12578

[110] Ozdeslika RN, Olinskib LE, Trieuc MM, Oprianc DD, Oanceaa E. Human nonvisual opsin 3 regulates pigmentation of epidermal melanocytes through functional interaction with melanocortin 1 receptor. Proceedings of the National Academy of Sciences of the United States of America. 2019;**116**:11508-11517. DOI: 10.1073/pnas.1902825116

[111] Cohen L, Brodsky MA, Zubair R, Kohli I, Hamzavi I, Sadeghpour M. Cutaneous interaction with visible light: What do we know. Journal of the American Academy of Dermatology. 2020. DOI: 10.1016/j.jaad.2020.03.115. PMID: 32289393 [Epub ahead of print]

[112] Fatima S, Braunberger T, Mohammad TF, Kohli I, Hamzavi IH. The role of sunscreen in melasma and postinflammatory hyperpigmentation. Indian Journal of Dermatology. 2020;**65**:5-10. DOI: 10.4103/ijd.IJD_295_18

[113] Praetorius C, Strum RA, Steingrimsson E. Sun-induced freckling: Ephelides and solar lentigines. Pigment Cell & Melanoma Research. 2014;**27**: 339-350. DOI: 10.1111/pcmr.12232

[114] Castanedo-Cazares JP, Hernandez-Blanco D, Carlos-Ortega B, Fuentes-Ahumada C, Torres-Álvarez B. Near-visible light and UV photoprotection in the treatment of melasma: A double-blind randomized trial. Photodermatology, Photoimmunology & Photomedicine. 2014;**30**:35-42. DOI: 10.1111/phpp.12086

[115] Boukari F, Jourdan E, Fontas E, Montaudié H, Castela E, Lacour JP, et al. Prevention of melasma relapses with sunscreen combining protection against UV and short wavelengths of visible light: A prospective randomized comparative trial. Journal of the American Academy of Dermatology. 2015;**72**:189-190. DOI: 10.1016/j.jaad.2014.08.023

[116] Geisler AN, Austin E, Nguyen J, Hamzavi I, Jagdeo J, Lim HW. Visible light part II. Photoprotection against visible and ultraviolet light. Journal of the American Academy of Dermatology. 2021;**84**:1233-1244. DOI: 10.1016/j.jaad.2020.11.074

[117] Halder RM, Richards GM. Management of dyschromias in ethnic skin. Dermatologic Therapy. 2004;**17**: 151-157. DOI: 10.1111/j.1396-0296.2004.04015.x

[118] Levitt J. The safety of hydroquinone: A dermatologist's response to the 2006 Federal Register. Journal of the American Academy of Dermatology. 2007;**57**:854-872. DOI: 10.1016/j.jaad.2007.02.020

[119] Schwartz C, Jan A, and Zito PM. Hydroquinone. In: StatPearls. Treasure Island, FL: StatPearls Publishing; 2022 https://www.ncbi.nlm.nih.gov/books/NBK539693/

[120] Gupta AK, Gover MD, Nouri K, Taylor S. The treatment of melasma: A review of clinical trials. Journal of the American Academy of Dermatology. 2006;**55**:1048-1065. DOI: 10.1016/j.jaad.2006.02.009

[121] Torok HM, Jones T, Rich P, Smith S, Tschen E. Hydroquinone 4%, tretinoin 0.05%, fluocinolone acetonide 0.01%: A safe and efficacious 12-month treatment for melasma. Cutis. 2005;**75**:57-62

[122] Chan R, Park KC, Lee MH, Lee E-S, Chang SE, Leow YH, et al. A randomized controlled trial of the efficacy and

safety of a fixed triple combination (fluocinolone acetonide 0.01%, hydroquinone 4%, tretinoin 0.05%) compared with hydroquinone 4% cream in Asian patients with moderate to severe melasma. The British Journal of Dermatology. 2008;**159**:697-703. DOI: 10.1111/j.1365-2133.2008.08717.x

[123] Chiari ME, Vera DMA, Palacios SM, Carpinella MC. Tyrosinase inhibitory activity of a 6-isoprenoid-substituted flavanone isolated from Dalea elegans. Bioorganic & Medicinal Chemistry. 2011;**19**:3474-3482. DOI: 10.1016/j.bmc.2011.04.025

[124] Chawla S, deLong MA, Visscher MO, Wickett RR, Manga P, Boissy RE. Mechanism of tyrosinase inhibition by deoxyarbutin and its second-generation derivatives. The British Journal of Dermatology. 2008;**159**:1267-1274. DOI: 10.1111/j.1365-2133.2008.08864.x

[125] Deri B, Kanteev M, Goldfeder M, Lecina D, Guallar V, Adir N, et al. The unravelling of the complex pattern of tyrosinase inhibition. Scientific Reports. 2016;**6**:34993. DOI: 10.1038/srep34993

[126] Smith CJ, O'Hare KB, Allen JC. Selective cytotoxicity of hydroquinone for melanocyte-derived cells is mediated by tyrosinase activity but independent of melanin content. Pigment Cell Research. 1988;**1**:386-389. DOI: 10.1111/j.1600-0749.1988.tb00140.x

[127] Arck PC, Overall R, Spatz K, Liezman C, Handjiski B, Klapp BF, et al. Towards a "free radical theory of graying": Melanocyte apoptosis in the aging human hair follicle is an indicator of oxidative stress induced tissue damage. The FASEB Journal. 2006;**20**:1567-1569. DOI: 10.1096/fj.05-4039fje

[128] Shariff R, Du Y, Dutta M, Kumar VS, Thimmaiah S, Doraiswamy C, et al. Superior even skin tone and anti-ageing benefit of a combination of 4-hexylresorcinol and niacinamide. International Journal of Cosmetic Science. 2022;**44**:1-15. DOI: 10.1111/ics.12759

[129] Mann T, Gerwat W, Batzer J, Eggers K, Scherner C, Wenck H, et al. Inhibition of human tyrosinase requires molecular motifs distinctively different from mushroom tyrosinase. Journal of Investigative Dermatology. 2018;**138**:1601-1608. DOI: 10.1016/j.jid.2018.01.019

[130] Nautiyl A, Wairkar S. Management of hyperpigmentation: Current treatments and emerging therapies. Pigment Cell & Melanoma Research. 2021;**34**:1000-1014. DOI: 10.1111/pcmr.12986

[131] Sanadi RM, Deshmukh RS. The effect of Vitamin C on melanin pigmentation – A systematic review. Journal of Oral and Maxillofacial Pathology. 2020;**24**:374-382. DOI: 10.4103/jomfp.JOMFP_207_20

[132] Boo YC. Mechanistic basis and clinical evidence for the applications of nicotinamide (niacinamide) to control skin aging and pigmentation. Antioxidants (Basel). 2021;**10**:1315-1339. DOI: 10.3390/antiox10081315

[133] Pullar JM, Carr AC, Vissers MCM. The roles of Vitamin C in skin health. Nutrients. 2017;**9**:866-893. DOI: 10.3390/nu9080866

[134] Huh C-H, Seo K-II, Park J-Y, Lim J-G, Eun H-C, Park K-C. A randomized, double-blind, placebo-controlled trial of vitamin C iontophoresis in melasma. Dermatologica. 2003;**206**:316-320. DOI: 10.1159/000069943

[135] Lee GSK. Intravenous vitamin C in the treatment of post-laser

hyperpigmentation for melasma: A short report. Journal of Cosmetic and Laser Therapy. 2008;**10**:234-236. DOI: 10.1080/14764170802187193

[136] Fuller BB, Spaulding DT, Smith DR. Regulation of the catalytic activity of pre-existing tyrosinase in black and Caucasian human melanocyte cell cultures. Experimental Cell Research. 2001;**262**:197-208. DOI: 10.1006/excr.2000.5092

[137] McGlinchey RP, Jiang Z, Lee JC. Molecular origin of pH-dependent fibril formation of a functional amyloid. ChemBioChem. 2014;**15**:1569-1572. DOI: 10.1002/cbic.201402074

[138] Miao F, Su M, Jiang S, Luo L, Shi Y, Lei T. Intramelanocytic acidification plays a role in the antimelanogenic and antioxidative properties of vitamin C and its derivatives. Oxidative Medicine and Cellular Longevity. 2019;**2019**:2084805, 14 pages. DOI: 10.1155/2019/2084805

[139] Chen S, Hseu Y, Gowrisankar YV, Chung Y, Zhang Y, Way T, et al. The anti-melanogenic effects of 3-O-ethyl ascorbic acid via Nrf2-mediated α-MSH inhibition in UVA-irradiated keratinocytes and autophagy induction in melanocytes. Free Radical Biology & Medicine. 2021;**173**:151-169. DOI: 10.1016/j.freeradbiomed.2021.07.030

[140] Lin H, Shieh B, Lu M, Chen J, Chang L, Chao C. A method for quantifying melanosome transfer efficacy from melanocytes to keratinocytes in vitro. Pigment Cell & Melanoma Research. 2008;**21**:559-564. DOI: 10.1111/j.1755-148X.2008.00487.x

[141] Ma H, Zhao G, Zi S, Li D, Liu W, Yang Q. Efficacy of quantifying melanosome transfer with flow cytometry in a human melanocyte–HaCaT keratinocyte co-culture system in vitro. Experimental Dermatology. 2010;**19**:e282-e285. DOI: 10.1111/j.1600-0625.2009.00956.x

[142] Greatens A, Hakozaki T, Koshoffer A, Epstein H, Schwemberger S, Babcock G, et al. Effective inhibition of melanosome transfer to keratinocytes by lectins and niacinamide is reversible. Experimental Dermatology. 2005;**14**:498-508. DOI: 10.1111/j.0906-6705.2005.00309.x

[143] Madaan P, Sikka P, Malik DS. Cosmeceutical aptitudes of niacinamide: A review. Recent Advances in Anti-Infective Drug Discovery. 2021; **16**:196-208. DOI: 10.2174/2772434416666211129105629

[144] Desai S, Ayres E, Bak H, et al. Effect of a tranexamic acid, kojic acid, and 509 niacinamide containing serum on facial dyschromia: A clinical evaluation. Journal of Drugs in Dermatology. 2019;**18**:454-459

[145] Ebrahimi B, Naeini FF. Topical tranexamic acid as a promising treatment for melasma. Journal of Research in Medical Sciences: The Official Journal of Isfahan University of Medical Sciences. 2014;**19**:753-757

[146] Ko D, Wang RF, Ozog D, Lim HW, and Mohammad TF. Disorders of hyperpigmentation. Part II. Review of management and treatment options for hyperpigmentation. Journal of the American Academy of Dermatology. 2022;**S0190-9622**(22):00252-00253. DOI: https://doi.org/10.1016/j.jaad.2021.12.065

[147] Mathapathi MS, Mallemalla P, Vora S, Iyer V, Tiwari JK, Chakrabortty A, et al. Niacinamide leave-on formulation provides long-lasting protection against bacteria in vivo. Experimental Dermatology. 2017;**26**:827-829. DOI: 10.1111/exd.13285

[148] Tanno O, Ota Y, Kitamura N, Katsube T, Inoue S. Nicotinamide increases biosynthesis of ceramides as well as other stratum corneum lipids to improve the epidermal permeability barrier. The British Journal of Dermatology. 2000;**143**:524-531. DOI: 10.1111/j.1365-2133.2000.03705.x

[149] Ahn KS, Moon KY, Lee J, Kim YS. Downregulation of NFkappaB activation in human keratinocytes by melanogenic inhibitors. Journal of Dermatological Science. 2003;**31**:193-201. DOI: 10.1016/s0923-1811(03)00039-2

[150] Bissett DL, Miyamoto K, Sun P, Li J, Berge CA. Topical niacinamide reduces yellowing, wrinkling, red blotchiness, and hyperpigmented spots in aging facial skin. International Journal of Cosmetic Science. 2004;**26**:231-238. DOI: 10.1111/j.1467-2494.2004.00228.x

[151] Hakozaki T, Minwalla L, Zhuang J, Chhoa M, Matsubara A, Miyamoto K, et al. The effect of niacinamide on reducing cutaneous pigmentation and suppression of melanosome transfer. The British Journal of Dermatology. 2002;**147**:20-31. DOI: 10.1046/j.1365-2133.2002.04834.x

[152] Navarrete-Solís J, Castanedo-Cázares JP, Torres-Álvarez B, Oros-Ovalle C, Fuentes-Ahumada C, González FJ, et al. Double-blind, randomized clinical trial of niacinamide 4% versus hydroquinone 4% in the treatment of melasma. Dermatology Research and Practice. 2011;**2011**:379173. DOI: 10.1155/2011/379173

[153] Khodaeiani E, Fouladi RF, Amirnia M, Saeidi M, Karimi ER. Topical 4% nicotinamide vs. 1% clindamycin in moderate inflammatory acne vulgaris. International Journal of Dermatology. 2013;**52**:999-1004. DOI: 10.1111/ijd.12002

[154] Damodaran A, Nair N, Shariff R, Damle A, Chandramowli G, Joshi P, Krishnamuthy H, and Vora S. Multiple modes of action of niacinamide in regulating skin pigmentation. In: Pigment Cell & Melanoma Research. 2014;**27**:849-1001. DOI: 10.1111/pcmr.12292. XXII International Pigment Cell Conference (IPCC); 4-7 September 2014; Singapore

[155] Castanedo-Cazares JP, Lárraga-Piñones G, Ehnis-Pérez A, Fuentes-Ahumada C, Oros-Ovalle C, Smoller BR, et al. Topical niacinamide 4% and desonide 0.05% for treatment of axillary hyperpigmentation: A randomized, double-blind, placebo-controlled study. Clinical, Cosmetic and Investigational Dermatology. 2013;**6**:29-36. DOI: 10.2147/CCID.S39246

[156] Engel K, Reuter J, Seiler C, Mönting JS, Jakob T, Schempp CM. Anti-inflammatory effect of pimecrolimus in the sodium lauryl sulphate test. Journal of the European Academy of Dermatology and Venereology. 2008;**22**(4):447-450. DOI: 10.1111/j.1468-3083.2007.02477.x

[157] Nair N, Dutta M, Karu J, Lim F-L, Damodaran A, and Logt P. Regulation of postinflammatory hyperpigmentation by niacinamide through potential modulation of the protease inhibitor, SERPINB3. In: Journal of the American Academy of Dermatology. 2022;**85**(Supplement):AB99. DOI: https://doi.org/10.1016/j.jaad.2021.06.417. Annual meeting of American Academy of Dermatology (AAD), 19-23 March 2021, San Francisco, USA

[158] Cork MJ, Danby SG, Vasilopoulos Y, Hadgraft J, Lane ME, Moustafa M, et al. Epidermal barrier dysfunction in AD. The Journal of Investigative Dermatology. 2009;**129**:1892-1908. DOI: 10.1038/jid.2009.133

[159] Kelhälä HL, Palatsi R, Fyhrquist N, Lehtimäki S, Väyrynen JP, KallioinenM KME, et al. IL-17/Th17 pathway is activated in acne lesions. PLoS One. 2014;**9**:e105238. DOI: 10.1371/journal.pone.0105238

[160] Hearing VJ, Jimenez M. Mammalian tyrosinase-the critical regulatory control point in melanocyte pigmentation. The International Journal of Biochemistry. 1987;**19**:1141-1147. DOI: 10.1016/0020-711x(87)90095-4

[161] Sanchez-Ferrer A, Rodrıguez-Lopez JN, Garcıa-Canovas F, García-Carmona F. Tyrosinase: A comprehensive review of its mechanism. Biochimica et Biophysica Acta. 1995;**1247**:1-11. DOI: 10.1016/0167-4838(94)00204-t

[162] Cooksey CJ, Garratt PJ, Land EJ, Pavel S, Ramsden CA, Riley PA, et al. Evidence of the indirect formation of the catecholic intermediate substrate responsible for the autoactivation kinetics of tyrosinase. The Journal of Biological Chemistry. 1997;**272**:26226-26235. DOI: 10.1074/jbc.272.42.26226

[163] Ramsden CA, Riley PA. Tyrosinase: The four oxidation states of the active site and their relevance to enzymatic activation, oxidation and inactivation. Bioorganic & Medicinal Chemistry. 2014;**22**:2388-2395. DOI: 10.1016/j.bmc.2014.02.048

[164] Zolghadri S, Bahrami A, Hasan KhanMT,Munoz-MunozJ,Garcia-MolinaF, Garcia-Canovas F, et al. A comprehensive review on tyrosinase inhibitors. Journal of Enzyme Inhibition and Medicinal Chemistry. 2019;**34**(1):279-309. DOI: 10.1080/14756366.2018.1545767

[165] Pillaiyar T, Manickam M, Namasivayam V. Skin whitening agents: Medicinal chemistry perspective of tyrosinase inhibitors. Journal of Enzyme Inhibition and Medicinal Chemistry. 2017;**32**:403-425. DOI: 10.1080/14756366.2016.1256882

[166] Espin JC, Varon R, Fenoll LG, Gilabert MA, García-Ruíz PA, Tudela J, et al. Kinetic characterization of the substrate specificity and mechanism of mushroom tyrosinase. European Journal of Biochemistry. 2000;**267**:1270-1279. DOI: 10.1046/j.1432-1327.2000.01013.x

[167] Muñoz-Muñoz JL, Acosta-Motos JR, Garcia-Molina F, Varon R, Garcia-Ruíz PA, Tudela J, et al. Tyrosinase inactivation in its action on dopa. Biochimica et Biophysica Acta. 2010;**1804**:1467-1475. DOI: 10.1016/j.bbapap.2010.02.015

[168] Mann T, Scherner C, Rohm KH, Kolbe L. Structure-activity relationships of thiazolyl resorcinols, potent and selective inhibitors of human tyrosinase. International Journal of Molecular Sciences. 2018;**19**:690-704. DOI: 10.3390/ijms19030690

[169] Stratford MRL, Ramsden CA, Riley PA. Mechanistic studies of the inactivation of tyrosinase by resorcinol. Bioorganic & Medicinal Chemistry. 2013;**21**:1166-1173. DOI: 10.1016/j.bmc.2012.12.031

[170] Shimizu K, Kondo R, Sakai K. Inhibition of tyrosinase by flavonoids, stilbenes and related 4-substituted resorcinols: Structure activity investigations. Planta Medica. 2000;**66**:11-15. DOI: 10.1055/s-2000-11113

[171] Schmaus G, Vielhaber G, Jacobs K, Franke H. 4-(1-Phenylethyl) 1,3-benzenediol: A new highly potent lightening agent. Journal of Cosmetic Science. 2006;**57**:197-198

[172] Vielhaber G, Schmaus G, Jacobs K, Franke H, Lange S, Herrmann M, et al.

4-(1-Phenylethyl)1,3-benzenediol: A new, highly efficient lightening agent. International Journal of Cosmetic Science. 2007;**29**:63-65. DOI: 10.1111/j.1467-2494.2007.00355_6.x

[173] Kolbe L, Mann T, Gerwat W, Batzer J, Ahlheit S, Scherner C, et al. 4-n-butylresorcinol, a highly effective tyrosinase inhibitor for the topical treatment of hyperpigmentation. Journal of the European Academy of Dermatology and Venereology. 2013;**27**:19-23. DOI: 10.1111/jdv.12051

[174] Limsuwan T, Boonme P, Khongkow P, Amnuaikit T. Ethosomes of phenylethyl resorcinol as vesicular delivery system for skin lightening applications. Biomedical Research. 2017;**2017**:8310979. DOI: 10.1155/2017/8310979

[175] Fan H, Li Y, Huang Y, Liu G, and Xia Q. Preparation and evaluation of phenylethyl resorcinol liposome. Integrated Ferroelectrics 2014;**151**: 89-98. DOI: https://doi.org/10.1080/10584587.2014.899873

[176] Kim DS, Kim SY, Park SH, Choi YG, Kwon SB, Kim MK, et al. Inhibitory effects of 4-n-butylresorcinol on tyrosinase activity and melanin synthesis. Biological & Pharmaceutical Bulletin. 2005;**28**:2216-2219. DOI: 10.1248/bpb.28.2216

[177] Huh SY, Shin JW, Na J, Huh C, Youn S, Park K. The efficacy and safety of 4-n-butylresorcinol 0.1% cream for the treatment of melasma: A randomized controlled split-face trial. Annals of Dermatology. 2010;**22**(1):21-25. DOI: 10.5021/ad.2010.22.1.21

[178] Huh SY, Shin JW, Na J, Huh C, Youn S, Park K. Efficacy and safety of liposome-encapsulated 4-n-butylresorcinol 0.1% cream for the treatment of melasma: A randomized controlled split-face trial. The Journal of Dermatology. 2010;**37**:311-315. DOI: 10.1111/j.1346-8138.2010.00787.x

[179] Mohan MT, Gowda A, Jaiswal AK, Sharath Kumar BC, Shilpashree P, Gangaboraiah B, et al. Assessment of efficacy, safety, and tolerability of 4-n-butylresorcinol 0.3% cream: An Indian multicentric study on melasma. Clinical, Cosmetic and Investigational Dermatology. 2016;**9**:21-27. DOI: 10.2147/CCID.S89451

[180] Khemis A, Kaiafa A, Queille-Roussel C, Duteil L, Ortonne JP. Evaluation of efficacy and safety of rucinol serum in patients with melasma: A randomized controlled trial. The British Journal of Dermatology. 2007;**156**:997-1004. DOI: 10.1111/j.1365-2133.2007.07814.x

[181] Chang TS. An updated review of tyrosinase inhibitors. International Journal of Molecular Sciences. 2009;**10**:2440-2475. DOI: 10.3390/ijms10062440

[182] Makino ET, Mehta RC, Banga A, Jain P, Sigler ML, Sonti S. Evaluation of a hydroquinone-free skin brightening product using in-vitro inhibition of melanogenesis and clinical reduction of ultraviolet-induced hyperpigmentation. Journal of Drugs in Dermatology. 2013;**12**:S16-S20

[183] Frankos VH, Schmitt DF, Haws LC, McEvily AJ, Iyengar R, Miller SA, et al. Generally recognized as safe (GRAS) evaluation of 4-hexylresorcinol for use as a processing aid for prevention of melanosis in shrimp. Regulatory Toxicology and Pharmacology. 1991;**14**:202-212. DOI: 10.1016/0273-2300(91)90007-i

[184] Kim SG, Lee SW, Park YW, Jeong JH, Choi JY. 4-Hexylresorcinol

inhibits NF-κB phosphorylation and has a synergistic effect with cisplatin in KB cells. Oncology Reports. 2011;**26**:1527-1532. DOI: 10.3892/or.2011.1436

[185] Fidalgo J, Deglesne PA, Arroya R, Ranneva E, Deprez P. 4-Hexylresorcinol a new molecule for cosmetic application. Journal of Biomolecular Research and Therapeutics. 2018;**8**:170-172. DOI: 10.35248/2167-7956.19.8.170

[186] Kaur S, Kizoulis M, Fantasia J, Oddos T, Bigot N, Galera P, et al. 4-Hexyl-1,3-phenylenediol, a nuclear factor-κB inhibitor, improve photodamaged skin and clinical signs of ageing in a double-blinded, randomized controlled trial. The British Journal of Dermatology. 2015;**173**:218-226. DOI: 10.1111/bjd.13747

[187] Chaudhuri R. Hexylresorcinol providing skin benefits by modulating multiple molecular targets. In: Sivamani RK, Jagdeo J, Elsner P, Maibach HI, editors. Cosmeceuticals and Active Cosmetics. 3rd ed. Boca Raton, FL: CRC Press; 2015. pp. 71-82

[188] Won Y, Loy C, Randhawa M, Southall MD. Clinical efficacy and safety of 4-hexyl-1,3-phenylenediol for improving skin hyperpigmentation. Archives of Dermatological Research. 2014;**306**:455-465. DOI: 10.1007/s00403-014-1439-9

[189] Arrowitz C, Schoelermann AM, Mann T, Jiang LI, Weber T, Kolbe L. Effective tyrosinase inhibition by thiamidol results in significant improvement of mild to moderate melasma. The Journal of Investigative Dermatology. 2019;**139**:1691-1698.e6. DOI: 10.1016/j.jid.2019.02.013

[190] Lima PB, Dias JAF, Cassiano DP, Esposito ACC, Miot LDB, Bagatin E, et al. Efficacy and safety of topical isobutylamido thiazolyl resorcinol (thiamidol) vs. 4% hydroquinone cream for facial melasma: An evaluator-blinded, randomized controlled trial. Journal of the European Academy of Dermatology and Venereology. 2021;**35**:1881-1887. DOI: 10.1111/jdv.17344

[191] Disphanurat W, Srisantithum B. Efficacy and safety of 0.15% isobutylamido thiazolyl resorcinol combined with hyaluronic acid vs 0.15% isobutylamido thiazolyl resorcinol or hyaluronic acid alone in melasma treatment: A randomized evaluator-blind trial. Journal of Cosmetic Dermatology. 2021:1-10. DOI: 10.1111/jocd.14031

[192] Philipp-Dormston WG, Echagüe AV, Pérez Damonte SH, Riedel J, Filbry A, Warnke K, et al. Thiamidol containing treatment regimens in facial hyperpigmentation: An international multi-centre approach consisting of a double-blind, controlled, split-face study and of an open-label, real-world study. International Journal of Cosmetic Science. 2020;**42**:377-387. DOI: 10.1111/ics.12626

[193] Roggenkamp D, Dlova N, Mann T, Batzer J, Riedel J, Kausch M, et al. Effective reduction of post-inflammatory hyperpigmentation with the tyrosinase inhibitor isobutylamido-thiazolyl-resorcinol (Thiamidol). International Journal of Cosmetic Science. 2021;**43**:292-301. DOI: 10.1111/ics.12694

[194] Vachiramon V, Kositkuljorn C, Leerunyakul K, Chanprapaph K. Isobutylamido thiazolyl resorcinol for prevention of UVB induced hyperpigmentation. Journal of Cosmetic Dermatology. 2021;**20**:987-992. DOI: 10.1111/jocd.13615

[195] Kang HY, Valerio L, Bahadoran P, Ortonne JP. The role of topical retinoids in the treatment of pigmentary disorders:

An evidence-based review. American Journal of Clinical Dermatology. 2009;**10**:251-260. DOI: 10.2165/00128071-200910040-00005

[196] Ortonne JP. Retinoid therapy of pigmentary disorders. Dermatologic Therapy. 2006;**19**:280-288. DOI: 10.1111/j.1529-8019.2006.00085.x

[197] Rivas S, Pandya AG. Treatment of melasma with topical agents, peels and lasers: An evidence-based review. American Journal of Clinical Dermatology. 2013;**14**:359-376. DOI: 10.1007/s40257-013-0038-4

[198] Kurlandsky SB, Xiao JH, Duell EA, Voorhees JJ, Fisher GJ. Biological activity of all-trans retinol requires metabolic conversion to all-trans retinoic acid and is mediated through activation of nuclear retinoid receptors in human keratinocytes. The Journal of Biological Chemistry. 1994;**269**:32821-32827

[199] Riahi R, Bush A, Cohen PR. Topical retinoids: Therapeutic mechanisms in the treatment of photodamaged skin. American Journal of Clinical Dermatology. 2016;**17**:265-276. DOI: 10.1007/s40257-016-0185-5

[200] Davis EC, Callender VD. Postinflammatory hyperpigmentation: A review of the epidemiology, clinical features, and treatment options in skin of colour. The Journal of Clinical and Aesthetic Dermatology. 2010;**3**:20-31

[201] Momosawa A, Kurita M, Ozaki M, Miyamoto S, Kobayashi Y, Ban I, et al. Combined therapy using Q-switched ruby laser and bleaching treatment with tretinoin and hydroquinone for periorbital skin hyperpigmentation in Asians. Plastic and Reconstructive Surgery. 2008;**121**:282-288. DOI: 10.1097/01.prs.0000293869.00522.ec

[202] Kimbrough-Green CK, Griffiths CE, Finkel LJ, Hamilton TA, Bulengo-Ransby SM, Ellis CN, and Voorhees JJ. Topical retinoic acid (tretinoin) for melasma in Black patients: A vehicle controlled clinical trial. Archives of Dermatology 1994;130: 727-733. DOI: https://doi.org/10.1001/ARCHDERM.1994

[203] Mohsin N, Hernandez LE, Martin MR, Does AV, Nouri K. Acne treatment review and future perspectives. Dermatologic Therapy. 2022;**35**:e15719. DOI: 10.1111/dth.15719

[204] Woolery-Lloyd HC, Keri J, Doig S. Retinoids and azelaic acid to treat acne and hyperpigmentation in skin of color. Journal of Drugs in Dermatology. 2013;**12**:434-437

[205] Callender VD, Barbosa V, Burgess CM, Heath C, McMichael AJ, Ogunleye T, et al. Approach to treatment of medical and cosmetic facial concerns in skin of color patients. Cutis. 2017;**100**:375-380

[206] Bulengo-Ransby SM, Griffiths C, Kimborough-Green CK, Finkel LJ, Hamilton TA, Ellis CN, et al. Topical tretinoin (retinoic acid) therapy for hyperpigmented lesions caused by inflammation of the skin in black patients. The New England Journal of Medicine. 1993;**328**:1438-1443. DOI: 10.1056/NEJM199305203282002

[207] Phillips TJ, Gottlieb AB, Leyden JJ, Lowe NJ, Lew-Kaya DA, Sefton J, et al. Efficacy of 0.1% tazarotene cream for the treatment of photodamage: A 12-month, multicenter, randomized trial. Archives of Dermatology. 2002;**138**:1486-1493. DOI: 10.1001/archderm.138.11.1486

[208] Grimes P, Callender V. Tazarotene cream for postinflammatory hyperpigmentation and acne vulgaris in

darker skin: A double blind, randomized, vehicle-controlled study. Cutis. 2006;**77**:45-50

[209] Tan J, Thiboutot D, Popp G, Gooderham M, Lynde C, Del Rosso J, et al. Randomized phase 3 evaluation of trifarotene 50 µg/g cream treatment of moderate facial and truncal acne. Journal of the American Academy of Dermatology. 2019;**80**:1691-1699. DOI: 10.1016/j.jaad.2019.02.044

[210] Adamus J, Feng L, Hawkins S, Kalleberg K, Lee JM. Climbazole boosts activity of retinoids in skin. International Journal of Cosmetic Science. 2017;**39**:411-418. DOI: 10.1111/ics.12390

[211] Hawkins S, Adamus J, Chiang C-Y, Covell E, O'Leary J, Lee J-M. Retinyl propionate and climbazole combination demonstrates clinical improvement to the appearance of hyperpigmentation and deep wrinkling with minimal irritation. International Journal of Cosmetic Science. 2017;**39**:589-599. DOI: 10.1111/ics.12412

Section 4

Pigmentation Disorders in Skin of Color

Chapter 8

Pigmentary Disorders in Black Skin from Pathophysiology to Treatment

Fatimata Ly

Abstract

Pigmentary disorders are frequent and more visible in patients with darker phototypes (Fitzpatrick's IV–VI). They also have an important psychological impact and are the cause of inappropriate cosmetic practices. Pigmentary disorders comprise a wide range of pathologies, and the pathophysiological mechanisms have evolved considerably in recent years. Pigment disorders vary in their clinical presentation from achromia to hyperpigmentation to hypopigmentation. Inflammatory dermatoses, such as acne, are often complicated by postinflammatory hyperpigmentation; psoriasis and lichen planus are accompanied by dyschromia. Some skin diseases, such as mycosis fungoides, have atypical presentations in the form of hypopigmented plaques. All these dyschromias have an important impact on the quality of life and are responsible for practices such as voluntary cosmetic depigmentation with products like dermocorticoids, hydroquinone and mercury salts, and various depigmenting products. This practice is at the origin of pigmentary disorders, such as exogenous ochronosis, lichen-like and lupus-like dermatoses, and periorbital hyperpigmentation. Therapeutic management is difficult and relies on chemical (peeling), physical (laser), and medicinal means (tranexamic acid); hence, the interest is in prevention through early diagnosis and the avoidance of favorable factors.

Keywords: postinflammatory hyperpigmentation, black skin, pigmentary disorders

1. Introduction

Pigmentary disorders refer to all alterations in skin pigmentation, which may be congenital or acquired. They may be hypo- or hyperpigmentation secondary or not to underlying conditions, most often inflammatory. These pigmentation disorders or dyschromias may also be manifestations of underlying systemic diseases. Postinflammatory hyperpigmentation (PIH) due to acne is defined as hyperchromic skin macules varying from brown to black affecting the face and/or body occurring after and sometimes during acne. It results from an overproduction of melanin following skin inflammation. It can occur on all skin types but is generally more frequent, visible, and persistent in phototypes IV–VI according to the Fitzpatrick classification [1]. In black skin, pigmentary disorders are frequent reasons for consultation [2]. Indeed, almost all pathologies can be complicated by dyschromic disorders during their evolution. Whether it is postinflammatory hyperpigmentation or hypopigmentation, the functional and esthetic repercussions are significant, and the impact on quality of life (QOL) is considerable [3]. Curative treatments are expensive and have a limited response; hence, the interest is in prevention based on the avoidance of risk factors, an early diagnosis and treatment, and photoprotection [4].

In this chapter, we will successively classify the different pigmentary disorders and describe the epidemiology and the pathophysiology of these different pigmentary disorders as well as the clinical and dermoscopic aspects. We will end with the treatment of pigmentary disorders.

2. Skin diseases according to the phototype

The vast majority of books devoted to the study of dermatological conditions are illustrated with photos of light-skinned patients. This makes it difficult for learners to identify these diseases in patients with black skin. The clinical and dermoscopic semiological aspects of dermatological diseases vary according to the patient's phototype. In addition, the therapeutic and evolution of skin diseases are different between white and black skin.

Indeed, the intense pigmentation on black skin can modify the clinical aspects. By example, the erythema appears less visible and had a shiny appearance [5]. The classical aspect of the malar erythema of systemic lupus erythematosus may appear as hyperpigmentation; in lichen planus, the lesions appear shiny with a silvery sheen [6].

Generally, in the inflammatory skin diseases, the pigmentary disorders are more visible. For the vitiligo, the contrast with the black skin leads to a negative impact on the quality of life and psychological impairment [7].

The systemic diseases, such as lupus, systemic scleroderma, dermatomyositis, and sarcoidosis, are different in clinical aspect; the dyschromia is in the foreground [8].

For tumoral skin diseases, the characteristics are different; for melanoma, the most common localization is on the palms, soles, or nail [9].

The basal cell carcinoma is very rare and is sometimes has a tattooed appearance. For squamous cell carcinoma, it is secondary to preneoplastic skin diseases (genetic, chronic inflammation, scare of burns, etc.) [9].

Generally, the bacterial, viral, and parasitological infections are not different in their clinical presentation. The modifications seen are more linked to the long delay of consultation or the impact of alternative therapeutic in the clinical aspects. Some infections such HTLV1 and associated diseases such as infective dermatitis are more prevalent in some geographical areas (Sub-Saharan Africa) [10].

Owing to some practices, such as skin bleaching with high-potent corticosteroids, the superficial fungal infections are widespread and localized on the face like tinea faciei [11].

Treatment may be different due to the inaccessibility of health facilities and certain drugs not marketed in low-income countries. In the majority of cases of chronic diseases, such as atopic dermatitis psoriasis and systemic and autoimmune diseases, the rate of loss to follow-up is very high because of the lack of therapeutic education.

3. Different types of pigmentation disorders

Pigmentary disorders in black skin are varied and arise from different mechanisms. They may either result from postinflammatory damage or constitute manifestations of the disease.

Type of pigmentation	Disease
Hypopigmentation	Psoriasis Systemic scleroderma Vitiligo Discoid lupus Eczematides Hansen disease Achromic mycosis fungoides Parapsoriasis
Hyperpigmentation	Postacne hyperpigmentation Rosacea Melasma Atopic dermatitis Psoriasis Acute lupus Lichen planus Exogenous ochronosis Lichen- and lupus-like hyperpigmentation of the articulations Periorbital hyperpigmentation Adverse drug reaction (ADR)
Hypopigmentation and hyperpigmentation	Poikiloderma Tinea versicolor

Table 1.
Classification of pigmentary disorders by appearance and etiology.

In **Table 1**, we list the main pigmentary disorders according to the hypo- or hyper-pigmented aspect and according to the nosological group.

4. Epidemiology of pigmentary disorders in black skin

The pigmentary disorders are very frequent in black skin, with prevalence ranging from 5.4% in Nigeria [12] to 19.9% in the USA [13]. In a cross-sectional study conducted in public hospitals in Durban, South Africa, the authors found than dyschromias are the third most common dermatologic diagnosis with a frequency of 8% [14]. The most common subtypes of pigmentary disorders found in this study include vitiligo, postinflammatory hyperpigmentation, and melasma. In our experience, at the Department of Dermatology, Hospital Institut d'Hygiene Sociale of Dakar, the frequency of skin diseases with pigmentary disorders was 34.67% (unpublished data). In a multicentric descriptive study conducted in Paris, France, among 1064 Afro-Caribbean people, the main motifs of consultation were acne and pigmentary disorders, which represent 8.4% [15]. Pigmentary disorders affect the women and the adult more. Indeed, the majority of the patients in the study were female (n = 229; 75.8%) [7]. The most common pigmentary disorders in terms of frequency are postacne hyperpigmentation and pigmentary disorders. The postacne hyperpigmentation is very frequent estimated to be in 87% and persistent for one year or more in 52.6% [16].

The prevalence of pigment disorders in psoriasis was 23.7% in a single-center prospective study from February 2018 to March 2019. This study included 459 patients, out of which 287 are men with a mean age: 49.9 years ($\sigma = 16.2$) [17].

In systemic scleroderma, the prevalence of pigmentation disorders was 36.8%. Hyperpigmentation and hypopigmentation can be diffused or localized in sun-exposed area [18].

During cosmetic skin bleaching practice, the pigmentary disorders are very frequently found in 84.5%, and they are variable: hyperpigmentation of the joints, exogenous ochronosis, and lichenoid dermatitis [19].

5. Pathophysiology of pigmentary disorders

5.1 Postinflammatory hyperpigmentation

Recently, Maghfour et al. [20] have focused on the pathophysiology of PIH with recent development. The melanocytes and the dermal fibroblasts are involved. The mechanisms implicated are the release of inflammatory cytokines and growth factors. Among the mechanisms identified, the following are worth noting:

- The increase production of arachidonic acid metabolites (leukotrienes LTC4 and LTD4, prostaglandins, and thromboxane) that promotes melanogenesis through an increase of tyrosinase-related protein.

- Inflammatory reactions and UV light exposure induce the production and upregulation of prostaglandins, which are considered as paracrine factors for melanocytes.

- Some receptors (the most common on the skin PGE-2 and PGF2-∝) activated by their ligands increase the dendricity of melanocytes, and then, the transfer of melanosomes is facilitated.

The mechanisms by NO production after UV light exposure also play a clue role in the upregulation of tyrosinase activity and tyrosinase related protein (TPR).

Another mediator of melanogenesis is histamine, which is released from dermal mast cell and mediated by UV irradiation. Recently, Nakaro et al. [21] have revealed the prominent distribution of dermal mast cells in PIH lesions.

Mast cells are implicated in another way by the secretion of IL33 that promotes the expression of microphthalmia-associated transcription factor (MITF) (microphthalmia) and thyrosinase related proteins involved in melanogenesis.

5.2 Systemic scleroderma

In systemic scleroderma, there is a dysregulation of CCN3, a matricellular protein implicated in angiogenesis and pigmentation regulation [22].

Some authors found a downregulation of this protein in melanocytes in patients with systemic scleroderma and pigmentary disorders.

6. Clinical aspects of pigmentary disorders

The PIH is frequent in many inflammatory skin diseases; the most common are acne, lichen planus, and psoriasis, but also in cutaneous infectious and tumoral diseases. Others autoimmune skin diseases, such lupus erythematosus, scleroderma, and dermatomyositis, are frequently associated with dyschromias, which can lead to misdiagnosis. Wood's light examination and dermoscopy help to assess the diagnosis showing the common signs in different pathologies.

In addition to the common dermatological conditions, there are other dermatoses that are secondary to the cosmetic use of depigmenting products. The pigmentary disorders that accompany these various conditions are the cause of inappropriate cosmetic practices.

We will consider successively inflammatory dermatoses, infectious autoimmune systemic dermatoses, and finally dermatoses associated with the use of depigmenting cosmetics.

6.1 Inflammatory and autoimmune skin diseases

6.1.1 Acne

For acne, PIH (**Figure 1**) is very frequent and has an important impact on the quality of life and is a frequent reason for consultation more than acne lesions [1]. The clinical presentation is polymorphous, and the adult women are often

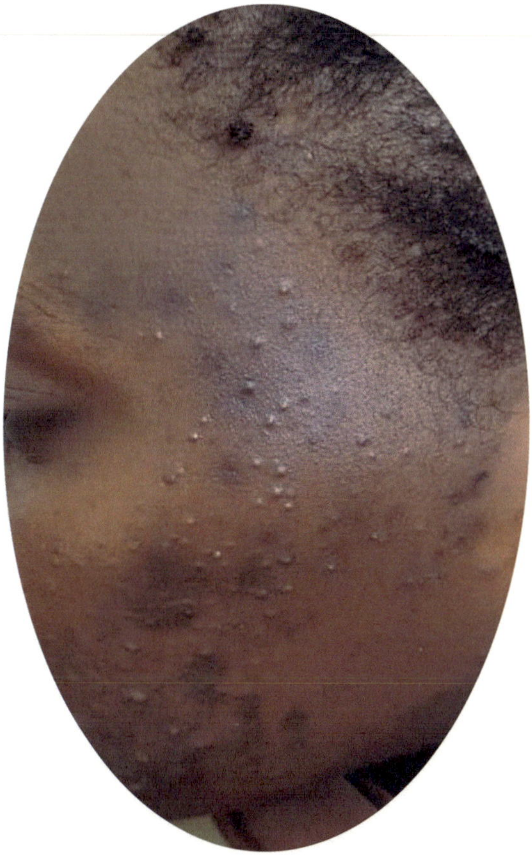

Figure 1.
Postinflammatory hyperpigmentation during acne.

affected [23]. A multicentric study had shown that PIH and involvement of the cheeks and forehead were significantly more common in darker phototype patients ($p < 0.001$) [24].

Pandaya et al. had already designed a scale to measure the severity of postinflammatory hyperpigmentation during acne [25]. This scale has been recently validated in phototype VI patients from Sub-Saharan Africa [26]. In addition to the severity of hyperpigmentation, this scale is useful for monitoring the evolution of the disease.

6.1.2 Psoriasis

Psoriasis can appear as lichenoid aspect, and dyschromias are frequently observed in psoriasis and may be either hyperpigmentation or hypopigmentation (**Figure 2**). Hyperpigmentation appears to be more frequent and occurs either in a lentiginous or diffuse form. Hypopigmentation has a well-limited border in the Wood's light [27]. These pigmentary disorders seem to be associated with an insufficient duration of treatment. It should also be noted that vitiligo can be associated with psoriasis [28]. The dermoscopic aspects showing the vascular aspect as globules and white squames help to assess the diagnosis.

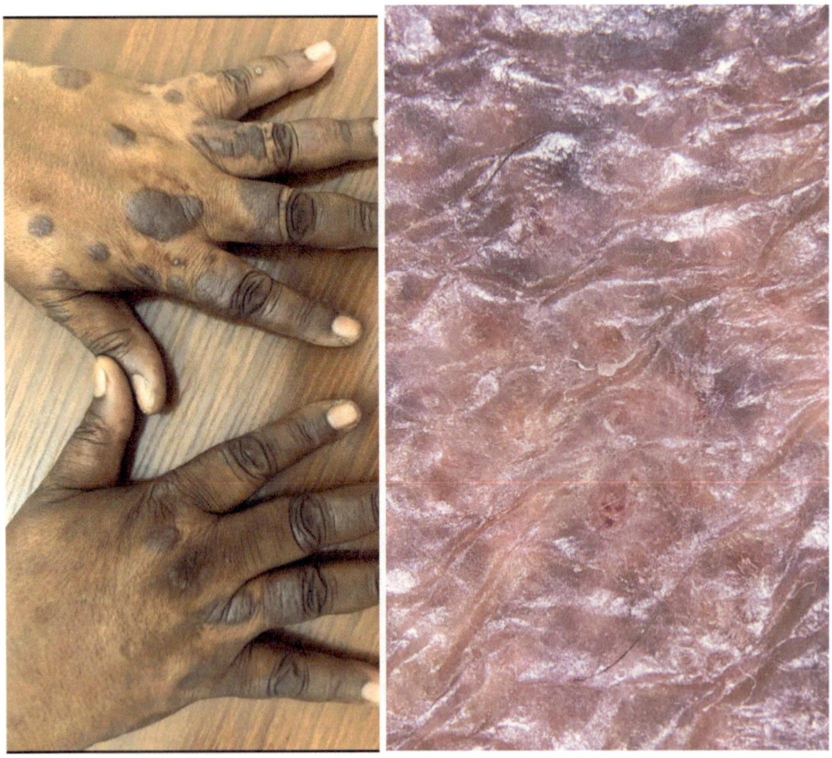

(A) (B)

Figure 2.
Clinical (A) and dermoscopic (B) aspects of psoriasis on the hand.

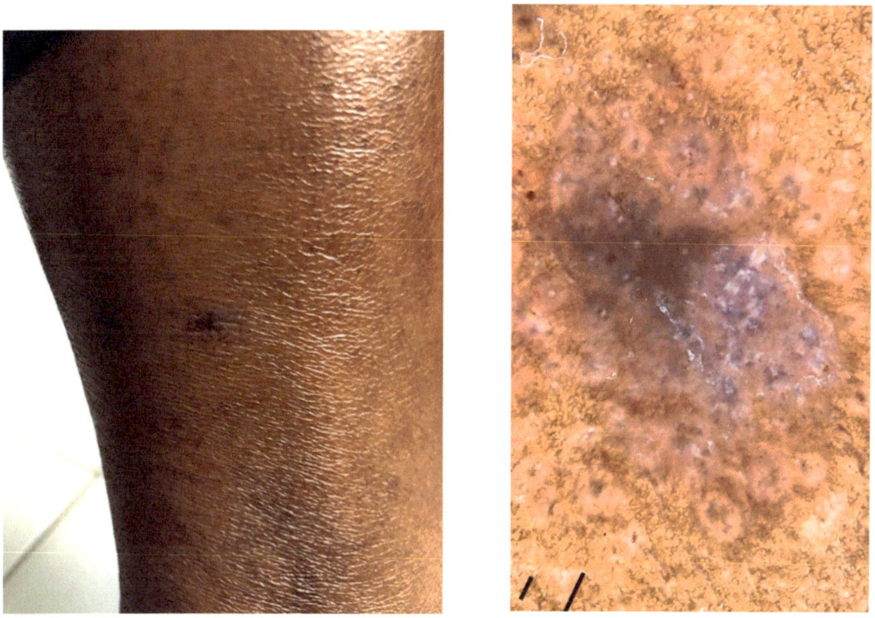

(A) (B)

Figure 3.
Clinical appearance with hyperpigmented (A) and dermoscopic papule with Wickham's streaks (B) of lichen planus.

6.1.3 Lichen planus

In patients with phototype VI, the lichen planus is characterized by pruriginous hyperpigmented silvery papules, which regress leaving large patches of hyperpigmented macules (**Figure 3**), which are unsightly. The topography is variable; the lesions may be localized or generalized sparing the face. No factors have been found to favor borderline or diffuse nature [29].

Clinical forms of pigmentogenic lichen planus have been reported in patients with a darker phototype. The dermoscopy is very helpful for diagnosis and to characterize the aspect of pigmentation, which can be homogenous or granular depending on the site of melanocytes [30].

6.1.4 Melasma

In black skin, melasma is a common condition more frequently seen in women, the etiopathogeny remains unclear, and many factors were incriminated: genetics, estro-progesterone, sun exposure, thyroid dysfunction, and pregnancy.

The clinical aspect is a brown or black macule localized on centrofacial, malar, and mandibular regions. Wood's lamp illumination shows epidermal (black or brown) or dermal (blue) pigmentation.

The dermoscopy shows scattered islands of brown reticular network with dark fine granules scattered on surface suggesting epidermal type of pigmentation.

In the dermal type of pigmentation, uniform skin involvement and no areas of sparing with dark brown gray hyperpigmented lesions with reticulo-globular pattern, telangiectasia and arciform structures [31].

6.1.5 Vitiligo

In patients with black skin, the clinical aspects with achromic macules on the skin and mucous membranes. Dermoscopy is useful to determine the disease's activity. Thus, perifollicular depigmentation (PFD) was predictive of stable vitiligo, and perifollicular pigmentation (PFP) was characteristic of active disease. Starburst appearance, altered pigment network, and comet tail appearance were also noted, and these were typical of progressive vitiligo [32].

Vitiligo is very stressful with psychological and emotional impact. Recently, in Nigeria, some authors assess the QOL impairment among Nigerian patients with vitiligo using a disease-specific quality-of-life index questionnaire (VitiQoL). They include 77 patients, and they found that QOL is impaired significantly in Nigerian patients with vitiligo [26].

6.2 Infectious skin diseases

The tinea versicolor can be associated in black skin with dyschromia [33]. Thus, macules may present as hyperpigmented or hypopigmented on the usual topography (**Figure 4**). However, in patients using high-potent corticosteroids for cosmetic purposes, clinical forms with achromic and atrophic lesions on the lower limbs may be found [34].

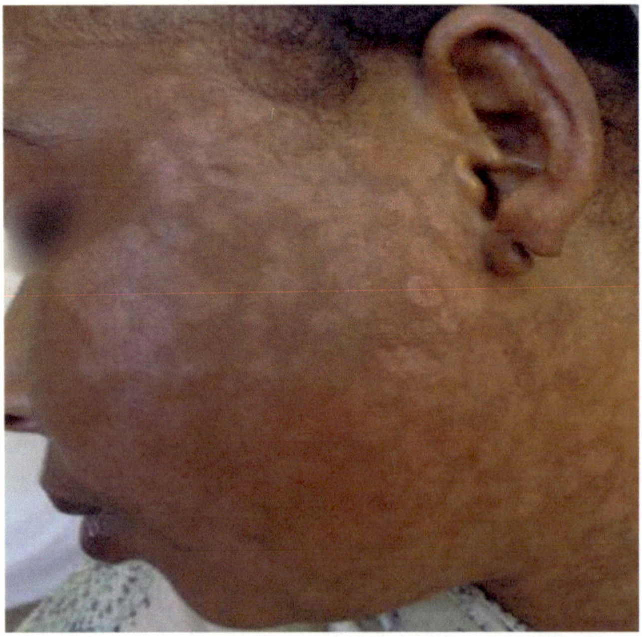

Figure 4.
Tinea versicolor on the face after skin bleaching by high-potent corticosteroids.

The clinical presentation of scabies varies with sometimes very diffuse hyperpigmented macules particularly in immunocompromised patients [35].

For other infectious skin diseases, the clinical aspects are variable: hypopigmentation is common in Hansen disease, in endemic treponematosis such Pinta, and in onchocerciasis. These latter are now very rare [36].

6.3 Systemic autoimmune diseases with skin manifestations

6.3.1 Lupus

In lupus, the dermatological manifestations are polymorphous; in patients with phototype VI, the skin disorders are often of pigmentary type (**Figure 5**). Whether it is specific acute, subacute or chronic lupus, or nonspecific, hyperpigmentation or

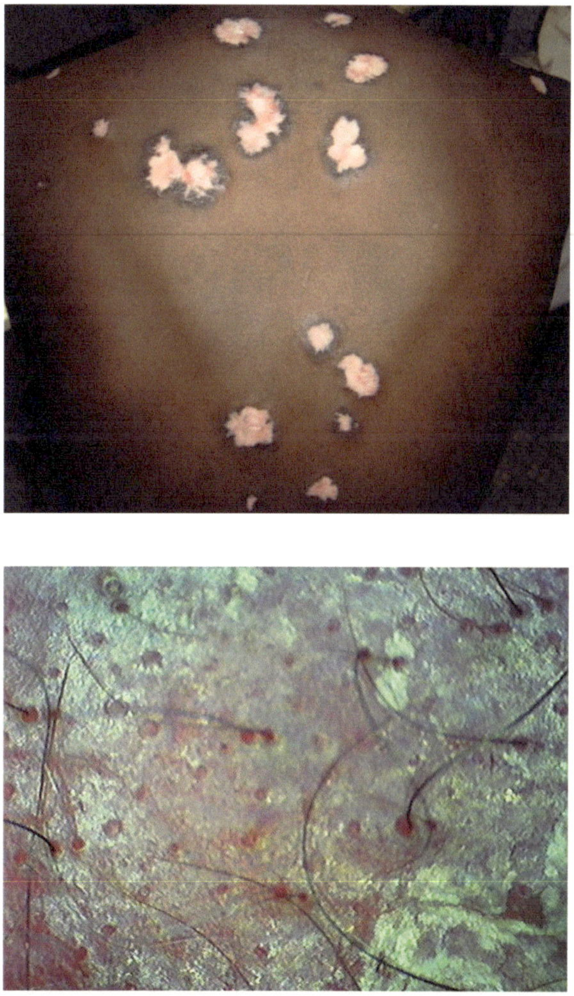

Figure 5.
Discoid lupus on the back clinical and dermoscopic aspect.

hypopigmentation is found in almost all the patients. For acute lupus, the vespertilio involvement may be complicated by hyperpigmented scars, depending on the intensity of the junctional involvement. For subacute lupus, it is more often the psoriasiform form that is complicated by hypochromia, whereas the annular form is rather hyperchromic. Finally, in chronic lupus, in addition to atrophy, erythema, and scaling, hypopigmentation is the hallmark. All these lesions have a considerable esthetic impact. Let us mention vitiligoid lupus, which is a variant of chronic lupus [37].

6.3.2 Systemic scleroderma

On black skin, scleroderma is characterized by pigmentary disorders, which are distinguished into five types. Hypopigmentation may be localized on the face, neck, and trunk (**Figure 6**), or on the extremities, or it may be diffuse, whereas hyperpigmentation may be either diffused or localized to the photoexposed areas [38]. The clinical aspects of pigmentary disorders during systemic scleroderma are the following:

- confetti depigmentation synonyms "salt and pepper," pseudo-vitiligo, speckled achromia, and speckled spots;
- diffuse hyperpigmentation;
- hyper- and hypopigmentation in areas of sclerosis;
- linear pigmentation within depigmented areas next to superficial vessels;
- localized hyperpigmentation;
- localized hyperpigmentation;
- Hyper- and depigmentation in belt with telangiectasia;
- hyperpigmented macules without cutaneous sclerosis.

Dyschromias are associated with the severity of the sclerosis. Indeed, diffused hyperpigmentation and hypopigmentation are more frequently found with a modified Rodnan score of over 30. The Rodnan score allows one to assess the degree of cutaneous sclerosis on different segments of the body (face, thorax, abdomen, and lower and upper limbs); it varies from 0 to 51.

Moreover, the duration of Raynaud's phenomenon of less than 10 years seems to be associated with the presence of dyschromic disorders.

6.3.3 Dermatomyositis

The particularities of dermatomyositis in black skin are flagellated macules and hyperpigmentation. Gottron's papules may take on a hypopigmented appearance. The association with muscular involvement helps the diagnosis [39].

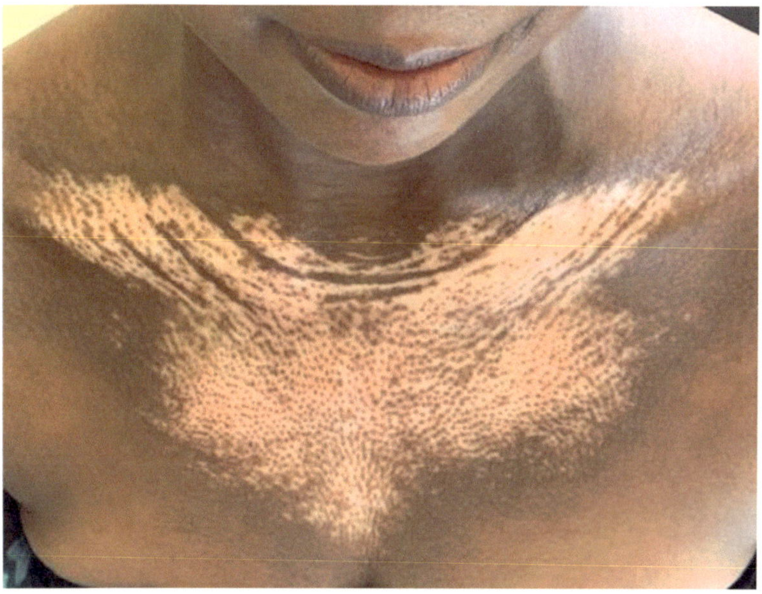

(A)

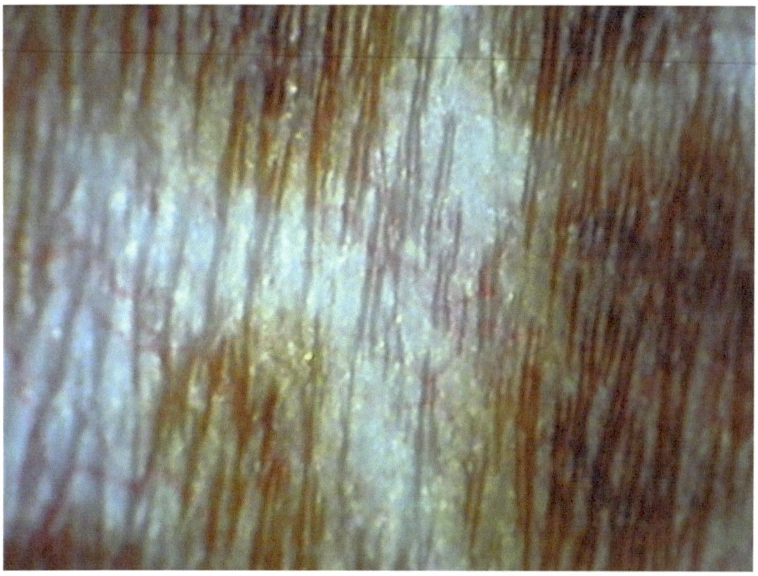

(B)

Figure 6.
Clinical (A) and dermoscopic (B) aspects of speckled achromia in systemic scleroderma.

6.4 Skin diseases associated with the cosmetic use of skin bleaching products

Skin bleaching is a practice consisting of the use of products containing high-potent topical corticosteroids, hydroquinone, and mercury or other depigmenting substances (fruit acids, kojic acid, arbutin, and injectable glutathione) for cosmetic purpose. It is a worldwide practice widely used by women from Sub-Saharan Africa,

Asia, and America. It is common in women from Sub-Saharan Africa where prevalence from 52–71% was found [40, 41].

The complications associated with this practice are varied, essentially bacterial, fungal, and parasitic infections, but also acne, trophic disorders, and pigmentary disorders. The latter include exogenous ochronosis, lichen- and lupus-like dermatoses, poikiloderma, and hyperpigmentation of the joints.

6.4.1 Exogenous ochronosis

Clinically, exogenous ochronosis is manifested by blackish papules with a tar-like appearance and a sensation of rape on palpation; these lesions are grouped in vast sheets and are located in the exposed areas (**Figure 7**). The back and the face are the most common localization, but recently other localizations have been described, such as hands on interdigital spaces and the backs of the feet [42].

6.4.2 Lichen- and lupus-like dermatoses

First described in 1976 by Marchand, the lupus- and lichen-like dermatoses are associated with a long-term use of hydroquinone.

The lesions occurred in a mean duration of 7.5 months after the use of hydroquinone and as macule or infiltrated papule with an annular border or hyperpigmented or macules (**Figure 8**). These lesions are localized on the face or upper limbs on the photoexposed area [43].

6.4.3 Poikiloderma

The poikiloderma associates atrophy, telangiectasia, and dyschromia and is secondary to the the association of high-potent corticosteroids and hydroquinone. The localization is preferentially on the upper limbs [44]. These complications are observed after a long-term use of bleaching products.

6.4.4 Hyperpigmentation

Hyperpigmentation can be localized or generalized; preferential localizations are the periorbital area or at the interphalangeal joints (**Figure 9**). This hyperpigmentation is one of the stigmata of skin bleaching.

This hyperpigmentation had a high psychological impact. Different types of pigmentary disorders can be associated in the same patient.

7. Treatment of pigmentary disorders

The treatment strategy of pigment disorders in patients with black skin remains a veritable challenge.

For symptomatic treatment, topical corticosteroids and retinoids are the most common treatment. However, hydroquinone at 4% alone, or in magistral preparations, gives a good result; arbutin and kojic acid are also indicated at all the stages of postinflammatory hyperpigmentation [42].

The photoprotection is also necessary for the treatment and the prevention of different pigmentary disorders.

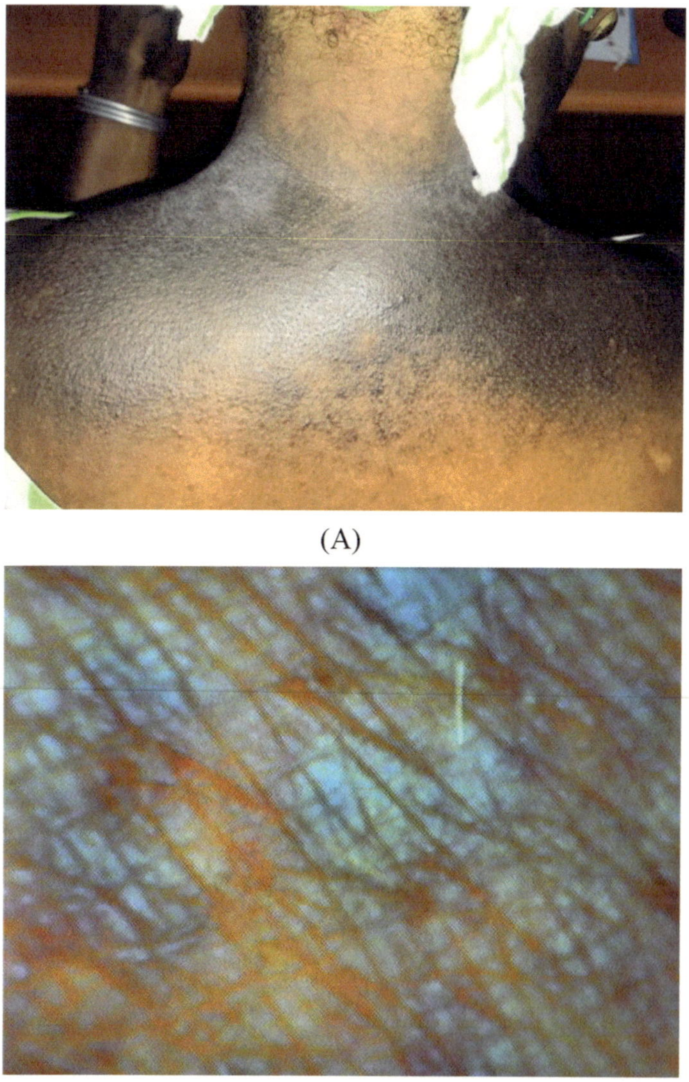

Figure 7.
Exogenous ochronosis on the back: Clinical with black papules (A) and dermoscopic aspect with brown gray globular structures(B).

For physical treatment, different types of lasers are available: 755-nm alexandrite picosecond, 694-nm ruby, and 532- and 1064-nm neodymium: YAG nanosecond lasers appear to be safe and effective modalities for the removal of pigmentary disorders in skin of color patients with no long-term complications if used appropriately [43].

For general treatments, tranexamic acid was used with good results in patients with melasma [44]. The early treatment of acne with low doses of isotretinoin, topical retinoids (adapalene), and photoprotection is associated with good results in acne postinflammatory hyperpigmentation.

For each disease, a specific treatment is indicated depending on the etiology and the patient's needs.

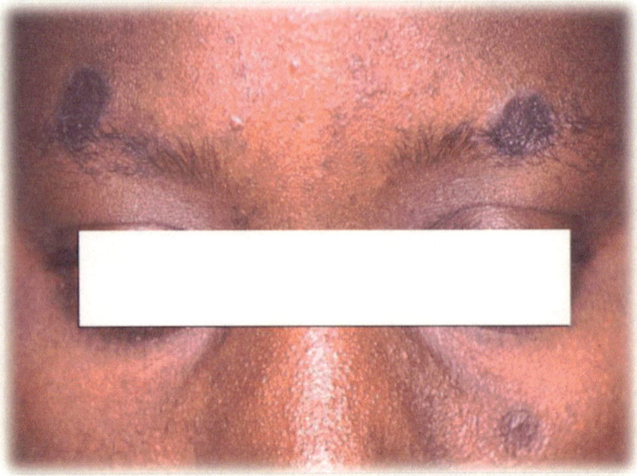

Figure 8.
Lichen-like dermatosis after skin bleaching with hydroquinone.

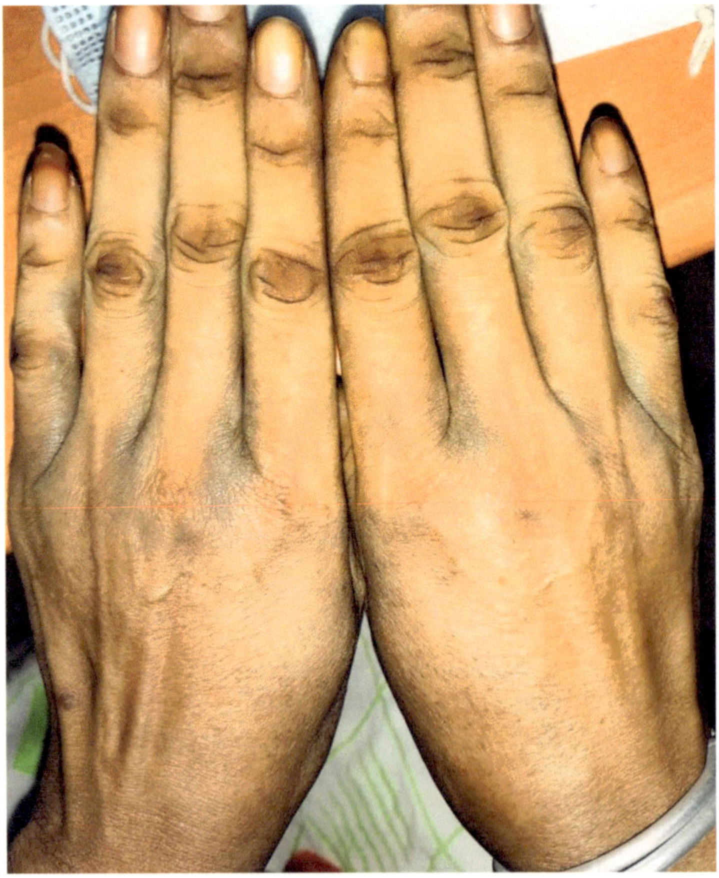

Figure 9.
Hyperpigmentation on the joints' dorsal aspect on the hand associated with exogenous ochronosis on interdigital folds.

Depending on the quality of life and the impact on pigmentary disorders, a psychological approach can be indicated [45].

Finally, prevention is particularly indicated in women using corticosteroids, hydroquinone, and mercury in cosmetic purpose. By information, communication and education by using safe cosmetics and by improving the cosmetovigilance system.

8. Conclusion

Pigmentary disorders are very frequent in phototype VI patient; etiologies are variables. Indeed, all the skin diseases can be associated with hyper- or hypopigmentation. The last few years' news data about the pathophysiology of postinflammatory hyperpigmentation were available. This latter is particularly associated with acne and can be evaluated by a scale that has been validated in phototype VI patients from Sub-Saharan Africa. The impact of pigmentary disorders on the quality of life of the patients with black skin was also evaluated. Moreover, dermoscopy, a noninvasive tool, is very helpful to establish the diagnosis and prognosis of such disorders.

The treatment is symptomatic and etiologic, and the prevention by photoprotection is a veritable challenge.

Conflict of interest

No conflicts of interest.

Author details

Fatimata Ly
Dermatology Unit, Institut d'Hygiene Sociale of Dakar, University Cheikh Anta Diop of Dakar, Senegal

*Address all correspondence to: lyfaty@yahoo.fr

References

[1] Chang MW. Disorders of hyperpigmentation. In: Bolognia JL, editor. Dermatology. 3rd ed. Elsevier Saundres; 2012. pp. 1052-1053

[2] Dlova NC, Mankhala A, Madala N, Grobler J, Tsoka-Gwegweni RJ. The spectrumof skin diseases in a black population in Durban, KwaZulu Natal, South Africa. International Journal of Dermatology. 2015;**54**(3):279-285

[3] Darji K, Varade R, West D, Armbrecht ES, Guo MA. Psychosocial impact of postinflammatory hyperpigmentation in patients with acne vulgaris. The Journal of Clinical and Aesthetic Dermatology. 2017;**10**(5):18-23

[4] Diffey BL, Fajuyigbe D, Wright CY. Sunburn and sun protection in black skin. International Journal of Dermatology. 2019;**58**:1053-1055

[5] Mahé A. Dermatologie sur peau noire. Paris: Doin; 2000

[6] Ly F. Psoriasis sur peaux pigmentées. Annals of Dermatology and Venereology. 2013;**140**:S11

[7] Parsad D, Sunil D, Jit KA. Quality of life in patients with vitiligo. Health and Quality of Life Outcomes. 2003;**1**(1):1-3

[8] Mahreen Ameem, Fatimata Ly. Cutaneous Manifestations of Systemic Diseases in ethnic Dermatology: Principles and Practice. 2013

[9] Dieng MT, Diop NN, Démé A, Sy TN, Niang SO, Ndiaye B. Squamous cell carcinoma in black patients: 80 cases. Annales de Dermatologie et de Vénéréologie. 2004;**13**:1055-1057

[10] Mahé A, Meertens L, Ly F, Sow PS, Diop CT, Samb ND, et al. Human T-cell leukaemia/lymphoma virus type 1-associated infective dermatitis in Africa: a report of five cases from Senegal. British Journal of Dermatology. 2004;**150**:958-965

[11] Mahé A, Ly F, Aymard G, Dangou JM. Skin diseases associated with the cosmetic use of bleaching products in women from Dakar, Senegal. British Journal of Dermatology. 2004;**148**:493-500

[12] Ogunbiyi AO, Daramola OO, Alese OO. Prevalence of skin diseases in Ibadan, Nigeria. International Journal of Dermatology. 2004;**43**(1):31-36

[13] Davis EC, Callender VD. Postinflammatory hyperpigmentation: A review of the epidemiology, clinical features, and treatment options in skin of color. The Journal of Clinical and Aesthetic Dermatology. 2010;**3**(7):20

[14] Ncoza C, Akintilo LO, Taylor SC. Prevalence of pigmentary disorders: A cross-sectional study in public hospitals in Durban, South Africa. International Journal of Womens Dermatology. 2019;**5**(5):345-348

[15] Arsouze A, Fitoussi C, Cabotin P-P, Chaine B, Delebecque C, Raynaud E, et al. Motifs de consultation en dermatologie des sujets de peau noire d'origine africaine et antillaise: enquête multicentrique en région parisienne. Annales de Dermatologie et de Vénéréologie. 2008;**135**(3):177-182

[16] Abanmi A, Al Enezi M, Al Hammadi A, Galadari I, Kibbi A-G, Zimmo S. Survey of acne-related post-inflammatory hyperpigmentation

in the Middle East. The Journal of Dermatological Treatment. 2019;**30**(6):578-581

[17] Amico S, Barnetche T, Dequidt L, Fauconneau A, Gerard E, Boursault L, et al. Characteristics of postinflammatory hyper- and hypopigmentation in patients with psoriasis: A survey study. Journal of AAD. 2020;**83**(4):1188-1190

[18] Leroy V, Henrot P, Barnetche T, Cario M, Darrigade A-S, Manicki P, et al. Association of skin hyperpigmentation disorders with digital ulcers in systemic sclerosis: Analysis of a cohort of 239 patients. JAAD. 2019;**80**(2):478-484

[19] Ly F, Soko AS, Demba Anta DIONE, Niang SO, Kane A, Bocoum TI, et al. Aesthetic problems associated with the cosmetic use of bleaching products. International Journal of Dermatology. 2007;**46**(S1):15-17

[20] Maghfour J, Olayinka J, Hamzavi IH, Mohammad TF. A focused review on the pathophysiology of post-inflammatory hyperpigmentation. Pigment Cell and Melanoma Resarch. 2022;**35**(3):320-327

[21] Nakano S, Abe Y, Nakajima K, Sano S, Yamamoto O, Wakamatsu K, et al. Establishment of a mouse model for post-inflammatory hyperpigmentation. Pigment Cell & Melanoma Research. 2021;**34**(1):101-110

[22] Henrot P, Pain C, Taïeb A, Truchetet M-E, Cario M. Dysregulation of CCN3 (NOV) expression in the epidermis of systemic sclerosis patients with pigmentary changes. Pigment Cell and Melanoma Research. 2020;**33**(6):895-898

[23] Kane A, Niang SO, Diagne AC, Ly F, Ndiaye B. Epidemiologic, clinical, and therapeutic features of acne in Dakar, Senegal. International Journal of Dermatology. 2007;**46**(SUPPL. 1):36-38

[24] Poli F, Faye O, Ly F, Le Thuaut A. Acné de la femme adulte: étude clinique en France et en Afrique sub-saharienne. Annales de Dermatologie et de Vénéréologie. 2014;**141**(5):336-345

[25] Savory SA, Agim NG, Mao R, Peter S, Wang C, Maldonado G, et al. Reliability assessment and validation of the postacne hyperpigmentation index (PAHPI), a new instrument to measure postinflammatory hyperpigmentation from acne vulgaris. Journal of the American Academy of Dermatology. 2014;**70**(1):108-114

[26] Khelife A, Diouf A, Diop A, Gueye FD, Mansouri H, Diousse P, et al. Reliability assessment and validation of the post-acne hyperpigmentation index (PAHPI) in a population from Sub-Saharan Africa in Senegal. Annals of Dermatology and Venereology. 13 Jul 2022;**2022**:S0151-9638(22)00059-X

[27] Alexis AF, Blackcloud P. Psoriasis in skin of color: Epidemiology, genetics, clinical presentation, and treatment nuances. The Journal of Clinical and Aesthetic Dermatology. 2014;**7**(11):16-24

[28] Yen H, Chi C-C. Association between psoriasis and vitiligo: A systematic review and meta-analysis. American Journal of Clinical Dermatology. 2019;**20**(1):31-40

[29] Diop A, Ly F, Ndiaye MT, Seck B, El Omari A, Diouf A, et al. Epidemiology, clinical features, and associated factors in 78 cases of lichen planus on black skin. International Journal of Dermatology. 2020;**59**(2):137-142

[30] Garcıa-Garcıa B, Munguıa-Calzada P, Auban-Pariente J, Argenziano G,

Vazquez-Lopez F. Dermoscopy of lichen planus: Vascular and Wickham striae variations in the skin of colour. Australasian Journal of Dermatology. 2019;**60**:301-304

[31] Sonthalia S, Jha AK, Langar S. Dermoscopy of melasma. Indian Dermatology Online Journal. 2019;**8**:525-526

[32] Degboe B, Atadokpede F, Saka B, Adegbidi HA, Koudoukpo C, Yedomon H, et al. Vitiligo on black skin: Epidemiological and clinical aspects in dermatology, Cotonou (Benin). International Journal of Dermatology. 2017;**56**(1):92-96

[33] Abdullahi U, Mohammed TT, Musa P, BO. Quality of life impairement amongst persons living with vitiligo using disease specific vililigo quality of life index: A Nigerian perspective. The Nigerian Postgraduate Medical Journal. 2021;**28**:169-174

[34] Kallini JR, Riaz F, Khachemoune A. Tinea versicolor in dark-skinned individuals. International Journal of Dermatology. 2014;**53**(2):137-141

[35] Mahé A, Ly F, Aymard G, Dangou JM. skin diseases associated with the cosmetic use of bleaching products in women from Dakar, Senegal. The British Journal of Dermatology. 2003;**148**(3):493-500

[36] Faye O. Diagnostic des hypochromies localisées sur peau noire. Annals of Dermatology and Venereology. 2006;**133**:877-884

[37] Diallo M, Diatta BA, Diop A, Ndiaye MT, Ndiaye M, Seck B, et al. Lupus erythematosus in Senegal: Study of 340 cases. Dermatological Case Report. 2006;**2**:135

[38] Diop A, Diadie S, Ly F, Ndiaye A, Ndiaye MT, SeckB DBA, et al. La sclerodermie systemique dans les services de dermatologie du Sénégal: une etude retrospective de 182 cas. Dakar Medicine. 2017;**62**(2):113-122

[39] Ndiaye M, Ndour N, Diadie S, Berrada I, Ndiaye MT, Sarr M, et al. Niang1 the profile of patients with Dermatomyositis in Dakar: A series of 56 cases Asian journal of research in dermatological. Science. 2021;**4**(4):23-29

[40] Ly F, Wone I, Ngom N, Fall F, Ndiaye MT, Diop A, et al. Epidemiology prevalence and factors associated with cosmetic skin whitening in the urban areas of parcelles assainies and Kaffrine (Senegal). Milan; 2019

[41] Ly F, Dangou JM, Ndiaye B, Mahé A. Dermatoses pseudo lichéniennes et pseudo lupiques secondaires à l'usage à visée cosmétique de produits contenant de l' hydroquinone. Nouv Dermatology. 2008;**27**:227-230

[42] Kaufman BP, Aman T, Alexis AF. Postinflammatory hyperpigmentation: Epidemiology, clinical presentation, pathogenesis and treatment. American Journal of Clinical Dermatology. 2018;**19**(4):489-503

[43] Jeremy MKLENYSCB, Brauer Roy A, Geronemus G. Treatment of pigmentary disorders in patients with skin of color with a novel 755 nm picosecond, Q-switched ruby, and Q-switched Nd:YAG nanosecond lasers: A retrospective photographic review. Lasers in Surgery and Medicine. 2016;**48**:181-187

[44] Virendra N, Srvastava S-PVG, Ashok K, Verma AS. Melasma: Treatment strategy. Journal of cosmetic and laser. Therapy. 2011;**13**(6):265-279

[45] Beresniak A, Auray J-P, Duru G, Aractingi S, Krueger GG, Talarico S, et al. Impact of pigmentary disorders on quality of life in Japan: Interest of the beauty QoL instrument. Journal of Cosmetic and Laser Therapy. 2015;**17**(6):313-317

Section 5

The Role of Melanin in Internal Organs

Chapter 9

Role of Melanin Pigment in Retina and Inner Ear

Donnell J. Creel

Abstract

Melanin pigment is normally present in the outermost layer of the retina of the eye, the inner ear adjacent to capillaries in stria vascularis near hair cells, and vestibular organs. Significant reduction in melanin pigment in mammals is associated with embryonic miswiring and disruption of visual and auditory functions. The consequences for the visual system include abnormal development of the retina and misrouting of optic pathways into the brain impairing visual acuity, eye movement, and stereovision. Lack of melanin pigment in the inner ear is associated with greater susceptibility to noise damage and poorer localization of sound in space.

Keywords: Albinism, melanin pigment, inner ear, retina, optic chiasm, stria vascularis

1. Introduction

The organization of the visual system varies among mammals. Most primates display well-defined retinal foveae, foveal avascular zone, and large numbers of uncrossed optic fibers at the optic chiasm. Mammals with laterally placed eyes, for example, guinea pig, rat, mouse, have little temporal retina producing few uncrossed fibers at optic chiasm. Cats and more so primates with forward-facing eyes have significant temporal retina, with nearly half of optic fibers remaining uncrossed at the chiasm of some primates. Mammals vary in proportion of optic nerve fibers that cross at the chiasm, embryonic development and optic projections terminating in vision centers from suprachiasmatic nuclei to midbrain, to geniculate nuclei, to visual cortex.

Most albino human beings and albino cats lacking retinal pigment have observable nystagmus and many exhibit strabismus. The optic chiasm of albino mammals including human beings and cats shows that almost all retinal ganglion cells cross at the optic chiasm with few uncrossed optic fibers. This misrouting has dramatic effects on organization of the visual system.

In 1965, C.L. Sheridan noticed that retinal ganglion cells originating in temporal retina of albino rats did not function well, hypothesizing that albino rats have fewer uncrossed, non-decussating optic fibers [1]. R.D. Lund anatomically verified that albino rats have fewer non-decussating optic fibers compared to pigmented rats [2]. For several years the abnormality of reduced non-decussating optic fibers at the optic chiasm in albinos was thought to be limited to rats and rabbits [3]. Guillery [4] reported atypical visual system organization in Siamese cats, but the association with albinism was not identified.

In 1971, Creel initially published the connection between Siamese cats and albinism, and hypothesis that reduced non-decussating optic fibers likely is a "highly general transspecies phenomenon in albino mammals" [5, 6]. Siamese cats, Himalayan mice, rats, and rabbits express a mutation that is a temperature-sensitive pigmentation defect, that is, allowing pigment only on the cold parts of the body. Their retinae lack pigment.

The studies of Siamese cat showed that a single recording site over each visual cortical area reflected differences between pigmented and albino cats [5]. Hence, scalp-recorded visually evoked potentials might detect optic misrouting in human albinos. Testing human albinos using scalp-recorded visually evoked potentials revealed human albinos have reduced non-decussating optic fibers [6, 7]. Animal studies reported that all albino mammals with oculocutaneous, or only ocular albinism, demonstrate reduced uncrossed optic projections [8–10]. Visual system abnormalities in albino mammals include fewer photoreceptors, foveal/area centralis hypoplasia, misrouting of the temporal retinal ganglion cells, variation of geniculate terminations, vascular intrusion into foveal area, abnormal cortical projections, and fewer cones in macular area [11–17].

The animal model close to organization of primate visual system studied the most is the albino cat. Albino cats have observable nystagmus, and many have strabismus. **Figure 1** pictures the optic chiasm of an OCA1 albino cat showing almost all retinal ganglion cells (RGCs) cross at the chiasm. The number of binocular cells is reduced in visual cortical areas 17, 18, and 19 in Siamese cats and albino cats impairing stereovision [19–21].

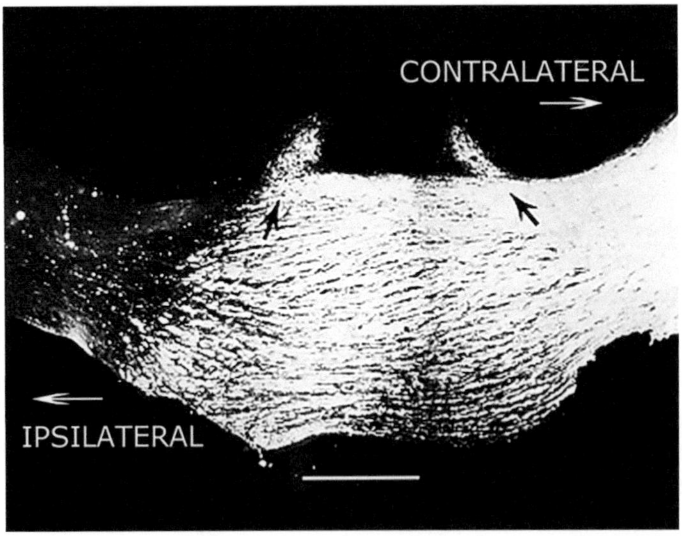

Figure 1.
Dark-field autoradiograph of coronal section through the optic chiasm of a Type 1 albino cat after injection of tritiated leucine into right eye showing difference between contralateral and ipsilateral RGC projections. Almost all RGCs cross at the optic chiasm. Arrows point to projections to suprachiasmatic nuclei. Scale bar 1 mm. From Creel et al. [18].

Phylogenetically older connections are less abnormal in albino mammals as seen in **Figure 1** showing bilateral suprachiasmatic projections appear to be unaffected [18]. Optic projections near chiasm projecting into hypothalamus antecede vertebrates, occurring in early chordates. Chordates have retinal pigment matching vertebrates [22]. Melanopsin retinal ganglion cells are completely crossed or bilaterally projected into suprachiasmatic nuclei above the optic chiasm [23, 24]. These projections are not affected by albinism. The crossed/uncrossed proportion of optic neurons to the suprachiasmatic nuclei in albino cats is like the proportion stated for pigmented cats [25]. The earlier appearing melanopsin pathway is not affected.

Abnormalities associated with hypopigmented retinae vary between species. Most human albinos have poorly formed foveae and little or no vascular sparing of central foveal area of retina [12, 26]. Visually evoked potential studies and functional magnetic resonance imaging reflect the preponderance of crossed optic fibers at the chiasm [15]. Few retinal ganglion cells originating temporal side of fovea in pigmented human beings cross at the optic chiasm. In albino mammals most retinal ganglion cells originating in temporal retina cross at the optic chiasm. **Figure 2** shows approximate differences between the optic chiasm of ocularly pigmented and albino human beings.

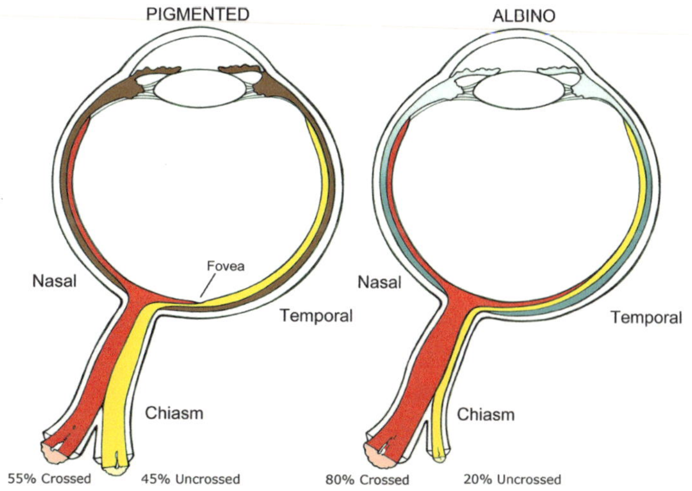

Figure 2.
Schematic of approximate distribution of crossed and uncrossed optic fibers in human beings. From Creel, webvision.med.utah.edu (2014).

Many possibilities are suggested for controlling embryonic retinal ganglion cells coursing through the chiasm. Some conclusions are likely to be correct within the model studied, but not a solution for optic misrouting seen throughout albino mammals. Each species varies. As an example, significant differences between mouse and human embryogenesis specific to chiasm formation are described [27]. Temporal timing of axon arrival at the optic chiasm and path through the chiasm are different between man and mouse. The development of contralateral followed by ipsilateral optic projections is sequential. There are no absolutes. Variable expression is seen even in littermate animal models [9]. Additionally, exceptions are reported [28, 29].

Due to millions of years of divergent evolution, the micro mechanisms of axon guidance underlying optic neuron decussation and target fate are likely idiosyncratic for each species. Pax2, Pax6, SOX2, and SOX21 seem to participate in development of the visual system. Several conserved loci including ROBO and PAX2/PAX 6 affect guidance in mammals including humans [14, 30–33].

Additionally, intra-genome communication is probably taking place. Visual embryogenesis is possibly affected by contributions from noncoding DNA and conserved noncoding portions of the genome. Noncoding DNA probably modifies expression [32, 33]. Variance within species appears to originate more in noncoding space [34].

Melanin is present in vertebrates and seen in early chordates. Melanin pigment is prevalent in mammalian embryonic development. Melanin pigment's function in the eye is different than in other parts of the body. Melanin pigment is present with melanocytes that are mostly active during early vertebrate embryogenesis. The melanin pigment chemical pathway initiated with tyrosine is expressed similarly from drosophila to primates. The sequence leading to eye formation in the fly is recapitulated in the developing human eye [35, 36]. Phylogeny is recapitulated in the embryonic development of the mammalian visual system.

1.1 Human pigmented vs albino visual system

Figure 3 shows OCT (optical coherence tomography) of the foveal area of a pigmented person (A) and an albino (B). In pigmented retina, the red nerve fiber layer does not cross the fovea. In most human albinos the nerve fiber layer (B) passes over fovea. Poor foveal development and variability among albino foveae are likely due to amount of ocular pigment and genetic background [37]. Albino human beings

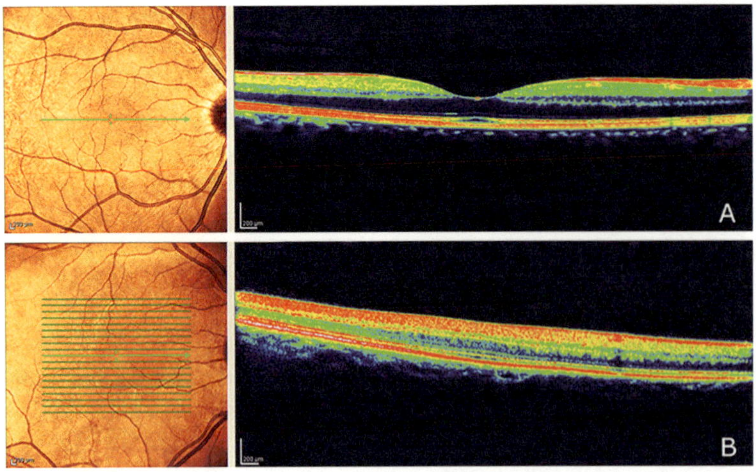

Figure 3.
Ocular coherence tomography (OCT) through the fovea of a normally pigmented (A) and albino (B) human being. Note the absence of foveal pit with the nerve fiber layer (red) continuing over foveal area in albino retina. From Creel, webvision.med.utah.edu (2014).

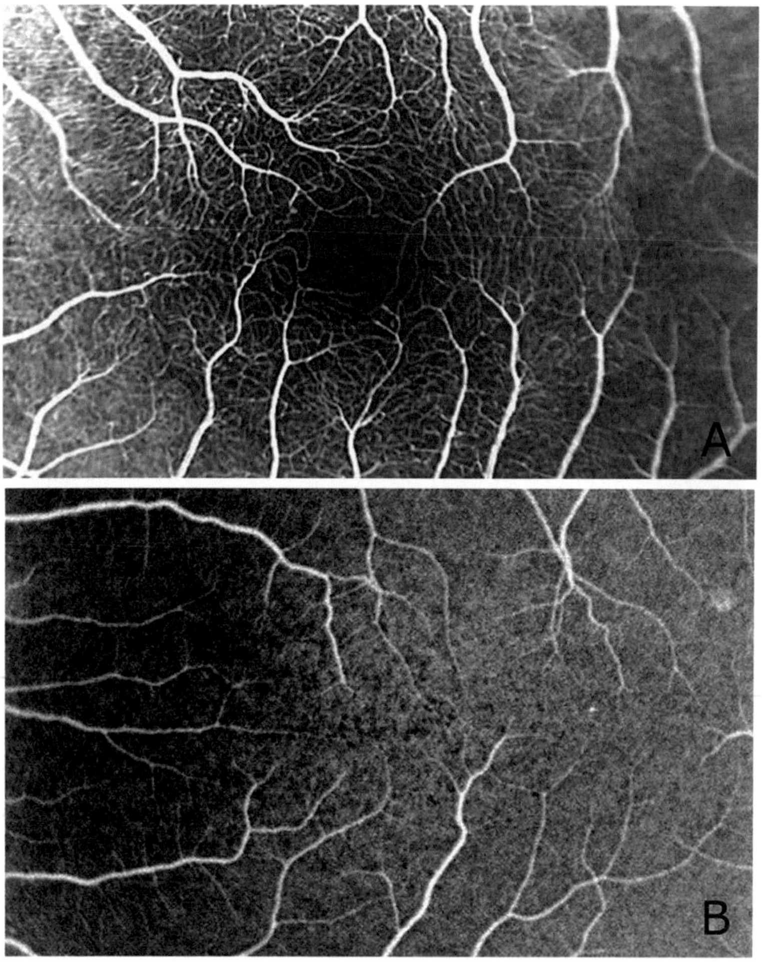

Figure 4.
Angiogram of pigmented human ocular fundus (A) showing vascular sparing of foveal area compared to albino (B) with vascular intrusion into vascular area. From Creel, webvision.med.utah.edu (2014).

manifest a reduction in cone density in the central retina [13]. Ocularly pigmented primates are the only mammals with developed foveae. In most mammals with albinism, the retinal macular area is underdeveloped [38, 39].

In humans with pigmented retinae, retinal blood vessels spare the foveal area. In albino human retinae, blood vessels intrude into foveal area. **Figure 4** compares the central vascular distribution in human pigmented and albino retinae. Pigmented humans exhibit an avascular zone surrounding the fovea. Albinos do not.

1.2 Pigment in inner ear

Vision and hearing evolved together dating back to the PaxB gene, which is a single gene controlling eye and precursors to hearing (mechanoreceptors) in box

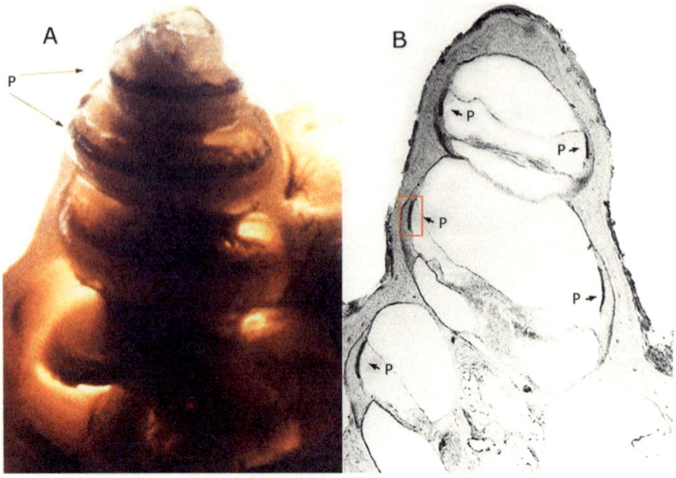

Figure 5.
Decalcified guinea pig cochlea (A) and sagittal section (B) through guinea pig cochlea show melanin pigment in stria vascularis. Red boxed area enlarged in ***Figure 6****. From Creel, webvision.med.utah.edu (2014).*

jellyfish before independent Pax 2 and Pax 6 genes [40]. There are evolutionary connections between eyes and mechanoreceptors of the inner ear to the extent that during evolution, "sensory cells can shift their sensory modalities" [41].

There is normally melanin pigment in the inner ear [42, 43]. **Figure 5A** shows band of melanin pigment (P) in a guinea pig cochlea. **Figure 5B** is a section through a guinea pig cochlea showing melanin pigment (P). **Figure 6** displays a microscopic view of area like that in red box in **Figure 5B**. Red arrows point at capillaries. Melanocytes are adjacent to capillaries in the stria vascularis of inner ear.

Binaural hearing tells eyes where to look [44, 45]. Spatial vision and auditory localization function in a coordinated manner. From diapsids to mammals interaural sound localization circuits are similarly organized. The auditory map in the brain is like the visual space map [46]. Visual and auditory space interact in the brain. When blind individuals localize auditory echoes, fMRIs reveal more brain activity in visual cortex than auditory cortex [47].

Albino mammals are not hearing impaired. The absence of melanin pigment in the inner ear is associated with susceptibility to noise damage [48–50]. Also, prolonged sensitivity to noise measured as a longer temporary threshold shift (TTS) following exposure to loud sounds is documented in albinos [51–53]. In the medial superior olivary nucleus, cell size and dendritic length are decreased in albinos [54]. In albinos component III of auditory brainstem responses is attenuated, which are generated in region of the medial superior olivary nuclei reflecting the reduced neuronal size and dendritic length in albino mammals [54–57].

The brainstem auditory pathways of albino mammals have anomalies like the visual system. Reduced cell size in brainstem olivary nuclei is associated with reduced binaural cell responses in medial superior olive of albino cats [58] resulting in disruption of sound localization, like finding of reduced binocular cells in visual cortex. Moore & Kowalchuk [59] described reduced ipsilateral projections from the cochlear nuclei in hypopigmented ferrets.

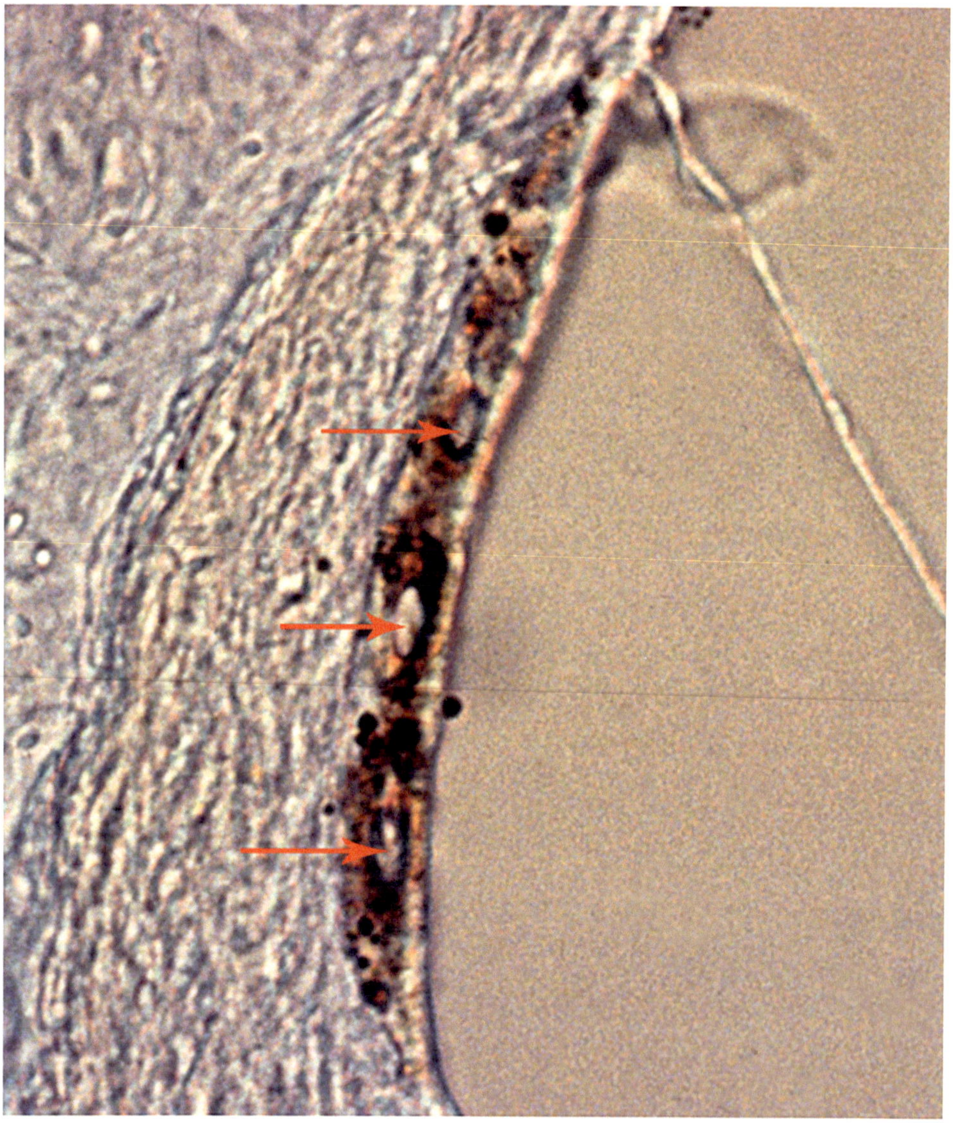

Figure 6.
Enlargement of red-boxed area in **Figure 5** *shows melanin adjacent to capillaries indicated by red arrows. From Creel, webvision.med.utah.edu (2014).*

1.3 Creel theory

The Creel theory proposes that the lack of melanin pigment initiates atavistic expression of visual and auditory embryogenesis. Melanin pigment is an environmental cue. Embryonic progression in albino mammals' visual and auditory systems take a step back initiated by lack of melanin pigment. Abnormalities of chiasmic misrouting in albino mammals is a developmental field defect that is normal in preceding phylogeny [60]. Complete crossing of optic neurons at the chiasm is normal in most vertebrates prior to mammals.

The presence of melanin pigment in the embryonic retina, or possibly genetic coding for melanin pigment, initiates retinal ganglion cell pathway routing. Insufficient coding for retinal pigment launches an earlier, more stable genetic package directing targeting of optic neurons.

Genetic makeup includes preserved earlier evolutionary features. Charles Darwin [61] popularized atavism as the term for reappearance of ancestral characteristics in future generations. Expression of atavistic features, such as complete crossing of optic fibers, is likely due to the flaw in the embryonic environment, in this case, lack of melanin pigment, precipitating formation of an earlier ancestral pathway.

2. Conclusion

Mammals lacking melanin pigment in retina and inner ear have abnormal visual and auditory systems. Mammals preserve the genetic instructions for complete decussation of the retinal ganglion cells at the optic chiasm and presence of melanin pigment adjacent to capillaries in inner ear. Phylogenetically newer genetic directions for formation of a central retinal area, fovea, and vascular sparing of the foveal area are vulnerable. Recent genetic addendums to conserved instructions are at risk if genetic cues, such as sufficient melanin pigmentation, are not present to support variation from ancient instructions. In albino mammals, the genetic instruction for visual pathways defaults to the simpler, more entrenched, platform. The auditory system follows with similar disarray.

Acknowledgements

Supported in part by an Unrestricted Grant from Research to Prevent Blindness, New York, NY, to the Department of Ophthalmology & Visual Sciences, University of Utah.

Author details

Donnell J. Creel
Moran Eye Center, University of Utah School of Medicine, Salt Lake City, UT, USA

*Address all correspondence to: donnell.creel@hsc.utah.edu

References

[1] Sheridan CL. Interocular transfer of brightness and pattern discriminations in normal and corpus callosum sectioned rats. Journal of Comparative and Physiological Psychology. 1965;**59**:292-294

[2] Lund RC. Uncrossed visual pathways of hooded and albino rats. Science. 1965;**149**:1505-1507

[3] Giolli RA, Guthrie MD. The primary optic projections in the rabbit: An experimental degeneration study. The Journal of Comparative Neurology. 1969;**136**:99-126

[4] Guillery RW. An abnormal retinogeniculate projection in Siamese cats. Brain Research. 1969;**14**:739-741

[5] Creel DJ. Visual system anomaly associated with albinism in the cat. Nature. 1971;**231**:465-466

[6] Creel DJ. Differences of ipsilateral and contralateral visually evoked responses in cats: Strains compared. Journal of Comparative and Physiological Psychology. 1971;**77**:161-165

[7] Creel D, Witkop CJ Jr, King RA. Asymmetric visually evoked potentials in human albinos: Evidence for visual system anomalies. Investigative Ophthalmology & Visual Science. 1974;**13**(6):430-440

[8] Sanderson KJ. Retinogeniculate projections in the rabbits of the albino allelomorphic series1. The Journal of Comparative Neurology. 1975;**159**:15-27

[9] Creel DJ, Giolli RA. Retinogeniculate projections in albino and ocularly hypopigmented rats. The Journal of Comparative Neurology. 1976;**166**:445-455

[10] Guillery RW, Oberdorfer MD, Murphy EH. Abnormal retino-geniculate and geniculo-cortical pathways in several genetically distinct color phases of the mink (Mustela vison). The Journal of Comparative Neurology. 1979;**185**:623-655

[11] Elschnig A. Zur anatomie des menschlichen albinoauges (Translated: On the anatomy of the human albino eye). Graefes Archivfur Ophthalmologie. 1913;**84**:401-419

[12] Fulton AB, Albert DM, Craft JL. Human albinism light microscopy and electron microscopy study. Archives of Ophthalmology. 1978;**96**:305-310

[13] Wilson HR, Mets MB, Nagy SE, Kressel AB. Albino spatial vision as an instance of arrested visual development. Vision Research. 1988;**28**:979-990

[14] Azuma N. Molecular cell biology on morphogenesis of the fovea and evolution of central vision. Nihon Ganka Gakkai Zasshi. 2000;**104**:960-985

[15] McKetton L, Kelly KR, Schneider KA. Abnormal lateral geniculate nucleus and optic chiasm in human albinism. The Journal of Comparative Neurology. 2014;**522**:2680-2687

[16] Bridge H, von dem Hagen EAH, Davies G, et al. Changes in brain morphology in albinism reflect reduced visual acuity. Cortex. 2014;**56**:64-72

[17] Ather S, Proudlock FA, Welton T, et al. Aberrant visual pathway development in albinism: From retina to cortex. Human Brain Mapping. 2019;**40**(3):777-788

[18] Creel D, Hendrickson AE, Leventhal AG. Retinal projections in

tyrosinase-negative albino cats. The Journal of Neuroscience. 1982;**2**:907-911

[19] Di Stefano M, Bedard S, Marzi CA, Lepore F. Lack of binocular activation of cells in area 19 of the Siamese cat. Brain Research. 1984;**303**:391-395

[20] Leventhal AG, Creel DJ. Retinal projections and functional architecture of cortical areas 17 and 18 in the tyrosinase-negative albino cat. The Journal of Neuroscience. 1985;**5**:795-807

[21] Kalberlah C, Distler C, Hoffmann KP. Sensitivity to relative disparity in early visual cortex of pigmented and albino ferrets. Experimental Brain Research. 2009;**192**:379-389

[22] Vopalensky P, Pergner J, Leigertova M, et al. Molecular analysis of the amphioxus frontal eye unravels the evolutionary origin of the retina and pigment cells of the vertebrate eye. Proceedings of the National Academy of Sciences. 2012;**109**:1583-1588

[23] Lucas RJ, Hattar S, Takao M, et al. Diminished pupillary light reflex at high irradiances in melanopsin-knockout mice. Science. 2003;**299**:245-247

[24] Hattar S, Kumar M, Park A, et al. Central projections of melanopsin-expressing retinal ganglion cells in the mouse. The Journal of Comparative Neurology. 2006;**497**:326-349

[25] Hendrickson AE, Wagoner N, Cowan WM. An autoradiographic and electron microscopic study of retino-hypothalamic connections. Zeitschrift für Zellforschung und Mikroskopische Anatomie. 1972;**135**:1-26

[26] McAllister JT, Dubis AM, Tait DM, et al. Arrested development: High-resolution imaging of foveal morphology in albinism. Vision Research. 2010;**50**:810-817

[27] Neveu MM, Jeffery G. Chiasm formation in man is fundamentally different from that in the mouse. Eye. 2007;**21**:1264-1270

[28] van Genderen MM, Riemslag FC, Schuil J, et al. Chiasmal misrouting and foveal hypoplasia without albinism. British Journal of Ophthalmology. 2006;**90**:1098-1102

[29] Poulter JA, Al-Araimi M, Conte I, et al. Recessive mutations in SLC38A8 cause foveal hypoplasia and optic nerve misrouting without albinism. American Journal of Human Genetics. 2013;**93**(6):1143-1150

[30] Kosmik Z. The role of Pax genes in eye evolution. Brain Research Bulletin. 2008;**75**:335-339

[31] Kidd T, Brose K, Mitchell KJ, et al. Roundabout controls axon crossing of the CNS midline and defines a novel subfamily of evolutionarily conserved guidance receptors. Cell. 1998;**92**(2):205-215

[32] Woolfe A, Elgar G. Organization of conserved elements near key developmental regulators in vertebrate genomes. Advances in Genetics. 2008;**61**:307-338

[33] Woolfe A, Goodson M, Goode DK, et al. Highly conserved non-coding sequences are associated with vertebrate development. PLoS Biology. 2004;**3**:e7

[34] Lee JT. Epigenetic regulation by long noncoding RNAs. Science. 2012;**14**:1435-1439

[35] Hanson IM. Mammalian homologues of the Drosophila eye specification genes. Seminars in Cell & Developmental Biology. 2001;**12**(6):475-484

[36] Kumar JP, Moses K. Expression of evolutionarily conserved

eye specification genes during Drosophilaembryogenesis. Development Genes and Evolution. 2001:406-414

[37] Dorey SE, Neveu MM, Burton LC, et al. The clinical features of albinism and their correlation with visual evoked potentials. The British Journal of Ophthalmology. 2003;**87**:767-772

[38] Hendrickson A, Troilo D, Possin D, Springer A. Development of the neural retina and its vasculature in the marmoset Callithrix jacchus. The Journal of Comparative Neurology. 2006;**497**:270-286

[39] Jeffery G. The albino retina: An abnormality that provides insight into normal retinal development. Trends in Neurosciences. 1997;**20**:165-169

[40] Piatigorsky J, Kozmik Z. Cubozoan jellyfish: An Evo/Devo model for eyes and other sensory systems. The International Journal of Developmental Biology. 2004;**48**(8-9):719-729

[41] Fritzsch B, Piatigorsky J, Tessmar-Raible K, et al. Ancestry of photic and mechanic sensation? Science. 2005;**308**:1113-1114

[42] Conlee JW, Parks TN, Schwartz IR, Creel DJ. Comparative anatomy of melanin pigment in the stria vascularis. Evidence for a distinction between melanocytes and intermediate cells in the cat. Acta Oto-Laryngologica. 1989;**107**:48-58

[43] Conlee JW, Gerity LC, Westenberg IS, Creel DJ. Pigment-dependent differences in the stria vascularis of albino and pigmented guinea pigs and rats. Hearing Research. 1994;**72**:108-124

[44] Heffner RS, Heffner HE. Visual factors in sound localization in mammals. The Journal of Comparative Neurology. 1992;**317**:219-232

[45] Feng W, Störmer VS, Martinez A, et al. Sounds activate visual cortex and improve visual discrimination. The Journal of Neuroscience. 2014;**34**(29):9817-9824

[46] Grothe B, Pecka M, McAlpine D. Mechanisms of sound localization in mammals. Physiological Reviews. 2010;**90**:983-1012

[47] Thaler L, Arnott SR, Goodale MA. Neural correlates of natural human echolocation in early and late blind echolocation experts. PLoS One. 2011;**6**:e20162

[48] Mujica-Mota MA, Schermbrucker J, Daniel SJ. Eye color as a risk factor for acquired sensorineural hearing loss: A review. Hearing Research. 2015;**320**:1-10

[49] Meyer zum Gottesberge AM. Physiology and pathophysiology of inner ear melanin. Pigment Cell Research. 1988;**1**(4):238-249

[50] Murillo-Cuesta S, Contreras J, Zurita E, et al. Melanin precursors prevent premature age-related and noise-induced hearing loss in albino mice. Pigment Cell & Melanoma Research. 2010;**23**:72-83

[51] Garber SR, Turner CW, Creel D, Witkop CJ Jr. Auditory system abnormalities in human albinos. Ear and Hearing. 1982;**3**(4):207-210

[52] Conlee JW, Abdul-Baqi KJ, McCandless GA, Creel DJ. Differential susceptibility to noise-induced permanent threshold shift between albino and pigmented guinea pigs. Hearing Research. 1986;**23**:81-91

[53] Barrenäs ML, Lindgren F. The influence of inner ear melanin

on susceptibility to TTS in humans. Scandanavian Audiology. 1990;**19**(2):97-102

[54] Conlee JW, Parks TN, Creel DJ. Reduced neuronal size and dendritic length in the medial superior olivary nucleus of albino rabbits. Brain Research. 1986;**363**:28-37

[55] Conlee JW, Parks TN, Romero C, Creel DJ. Auditory brainstem anomalies in albino cats: II. Neuronal atrophy in the superior olive. The Journal of Comparative Neurology. 1984;**225**:141-148

[56] Creel DJ, Garber SR, King RA, Witkop CJ Jr. Auditory brainstem anomalies in human albinos. Science. 1980;**209**:1253-1255

[57] Creel D, Conlee JW, Parks TN. Auditory brainstem anomalies in albino cats. I. Evoked potential studies. Brain Research. 1983;**260**:1-9

[58] Yin TCT, Carney LH, Joris PX. Interaural time sensitivity in the inferior colliculus of the albino cat. The Journal of Comparative Neurology. 1990;**295**:438-448

[59] Moore DR, Kowalchuk NE. Auditory brainstem of the ferret: Effects of unilateral cochlear lesions on cochlear nucleus volume and projections to the inferior colliculus. The Journal of Comparative Neurology. 1988;**272**:503-515

[60] Opitz JM. 2011 William Allan Award: Development and Evolution. American Journal of Human Genetics. 2012;**90**(3):392-404

[61] Darwin C. The Variation of Animals and Plants under Domestication. Vol. 2. London: John Murray; 1868